Seven Steps to Better Vision

Seven Steps to Better Vision

Easy, Practical & Natural Techniques That Will Improve Your Eyesight

Richard Leviton

East West/Natural Health Books

East West/Natural Health Books
17 Station Street
Brookline, Massachusetts 02146

ISBN 0-936184-13-2
Library of Congress Cataloging-in-Publication Data
Leviton, Richard.
    Seven steps to better vision: easy, practical & natural
    techniques that will improve your eyesight / Richard Leviton.—
1st ed.
        p.   cm.
    Includes bibliographical references and index.
    ISBN 0-936184-13-2 (paperback) : $8.95
    1. Behavioral optometry.   I. Title.
RE960.L48 1992
617.7'5—dc20   92-11485
                                      CIP

Manufactured in the United States of America

First Edition   135798642

Distributed to the natural foods trade by East West/Natural Health Books, 17 Station Street, Brookline, MA 02146 and to the book trade by The Talman Company, 131 Spring St. 201E-N, New York, NY 10012.

Cover and text design by Sara Eisenman
Illustrations by Kathy Bray

The tools, techniques, and suggestions in this book are not intended to substitute for medical advice or treatment. Any application of the ideas in this book is at the reader's discretion and risk.

Contents

Acknowledgments

The author gratefully acknowledges the
kind assistance and healing insight of
Robert-Michael Kaplan, O.D.,
and Cathy Stern, O.D.

Foreword

In the past, the likelihood of improving vision through eye exercises seemed dubious in light of negative views held by most optometrists and ophthalmologists. Is it really possible, without surgery, to effect changes in the eye, or even the brain, which will result in clearer vision? Will specific techniques, methods, and exercises produce faster or more dramatic results? Does an integrated or holistic approach bring about longer-lasting and more effective changes?

Ninety percent of vision occurs in the brain. The eye responds to both incoming light and control from brain centers. To maximize changes in the eye itself, it is best to harness as much of the body/brain/mind connection as possible.

Even as researchers, clinicians, and doctors are aware of the interconnectedness of the organs of the body, so various disciplines can be combined to provide healing for the eyes and vision. The holistic approach recognizes that our eyes and vision are influenced by all factors in our lives. The food we eat, the way we think, our degree of tension or distress, daily visual habits, purpose, intention, breathing, posture, attitudes, and the movement of our eyes collectively play a more powerful role in our vision than any of the individual components are able to achieve alone. Holism in action accepts that the whole is greater than the sum of the parts.

The truly integrated approach requires a holistic frame of mind. Your attitude toward the vision improvement process is more important than the combination of techniques you use. Just doing such exercises as palming the eyes or "walking in the blur" without eyeglasses can be very effective if aligned with breathing, an internal awareness of purpose, and a strong belief that your vision will be improved. Heretofore, no single book interfacing the multitude of elements comprising the whole has been available for vision practitioners, patients, and students of vision improvement.

Seven Steps to Better Vision is a most comprehensive presentation. Richard Leviton has masterfully compiled extensive knowledge and research to include these proven methods. This book offers a concise roadmap of information and routes to guide you through the many avenues available for healing your eyes.

The journey to better vision is a worthy one with rewards in personal growth as well as in vision improvement. For some, the results can be immediate. Improving my own vision using these methods, and watching others do the same, has been fulfilling and exciting.

Take the first step. Read this book, then patiently design your personal path to better vision. As you begin your quest, choose a skilled guide, either a behavioral optometrist, vision therapist, natural vision teacher, educator, or other therapist, to assist you in determining what will work best for your unique eye condition.

Improving your vision naturally by applying the principles of *Seven Steps to Better Vision* is now within your grasp.

Dr. Robert-Michael Kaplan, O.D., M.Ed.
Former Professor of Optometry
Author of *Seeing Beyond 20/20*
Vancouver, B.C., Canada

Part One:
The Art and Science of Vision

Exploring the Visual Pathway

Without my glasses, my eyes feel naked and vulnerable as they're examined by Dr. Cathy Stern, an optometrist practicing in Brookline, Mass. Glasses are so habitual for me they've become part of my face, as if permanently glued to the bridge of my nose. I joke that I wear my glasses when sleeping so I can see better in my dreams. I've worn them every day since early childhood.

In fact, I've had my present pair for 21 years with the original prescription intact, a fact few opticians like to hear. They're much happier when eyeglass and contact wearers order new, usually stronger, prescriptions and change their frames every couple of years. Thus I'm surprised when Stern, whose practice of "behavioral optometry" focuses on vision improvement strategies, says to me, "Did you know you could reduce your refractive error with a weaker lens and eye exercises?"

No, I didn't. In the years I've spent studying health it never occurred to me that poor vision could be remedied. No doubt like most of the estimated 134 million Americans who wear corrective lenses, I've taken them for granted, as a permanent fixture of living, like shoes.

I try to imagine myself not needing glasses, seeing the world without the mediation of a quarter-inch of bulging glass. Is it possible? "At your level of nearsightedness and at your age I could never promise you'd be able to drive without your glasses and improve to 20/40 or 20/20," cautions Stern. "But a 30 percent or so improvement is possible, and that's significant by anyone's standards."

Stern is one of a growing number of vision improvement advocates in the U.S. who say that it is indeed possible to see better without glasses. Using tools and techniques that range from high-tech biofeedback machines to eye exercises to nutritional supplements, vision therapists have helped hundreds of thousands of clients to see more clearly, as well as to more quickly and accurately take in information through the eyes.

Even a possible 30 percent improvement in acuity would no doubt surprise most of the 72 million Americans who underwent eye examinations in 1990. Nor is it likely to sit well with the optometrists who wrote out 60 million eyeglass prescriptions for them. Glasses or contacts are an unquestioned fact of contemporary life for over half of all Americans. And lenses are big business for the optometrists, too. In 1990 Americans spent over $15 billion on eye care and prescription lenses. Most of this was for glasses, but some 23 million people now wear contacts, about double the number of only a decade ago.

The incidence of nearsightedness, also known as myopia, among children is rising, especially as modern culture becomes increasingly dominated by near-point demands, such as working at a video display terminal (VDT). According to behavioral optometrists Hazel Richmond Dawkins, Ellis Edelman, and Constantine Forkiotis, authors of the vision manual *Suddenly Successful,* America is experiencing "an epidemic of nearsightedness." Recent estimates are that while only 3 percent of children aged 5-9 are nearsighted, among high school-age adolescents the figure jumps to 40 percent. By college nearsightedness affects 60-80 percent of the students. "The reason it has not caused alarm," comment Dawkins et al., "is that it's possible to make a myope's vision clear with prescription lenses. But lenses that only work on the symptom of nearsightedness are compensating lenses; they mask the serious nature of the condition."

From Spectacles to Contacts

Current vision problems may be approaching epidemic proportions, but humanity has long sought mechanical ways to improve sight. Western history credits a late 13th century Florentine monk, Brother Alessandro di Spina, as the first "optician" to fit corrective lenses into frames. He may have followed up a hint from England's philosopher and scientist Roger Bacon, who observed in 1268 that spherical bits of glass magnified letters and figures. Bacon's hint for posterity was that small fitted lenses might be useful "to old persons and to those with weak sight, for they can see any letter, however small, if magnified enough."

By the mid-14th century corrective spectacles had become popular among European scholars. These first eyeglasses used convex lenses made of transparent beryl and quartz to correct farsightedness. The thicker, bulging concave lenses for myopia didn't start appearing until the early 16th century, judging by Raphael's painting of Pope Leo X sporting what are surely corrective glasses for myopia.

Even the idea of contact lenses goes back centuries, to Leonardo da Vinci's description of an artificial lens that could be fitted over the white of the eyes. But it wasn't until 1887 that A. E. Fick, a Zurich physician, successfully fitted a pair of glass contact lenses on the eyes of a man with cancerous eyelids. And it wasn't until 1938 that American opticians developed the first clear plastic contact lens. By 1960, a Czech had patented soft contacts, while more recent innovations include "extended wear" styles that can be worn without removal for 30 days, bifocal contacts, and seven-day disposable lenses.

At the same time that optometrists (holders of a doctor of optometry O.D. degree who measure vision errors and prescribe corrective lenses) were perfecting corrective lens technology, ophthalmologists (doctors who specialize in treating diseases of the eye) were building a comprehensive scientific picture of how eyesight and vision work. Among the most remarkable if elementary observations they made is that only 10 percent of the visual process takes place in the eyes. The remaining 90 percent occupies the brain's optic cortex, located at the base of the skull in the occipital lobe. This means that sight is the result of a complex interaction along a visual pathway that extends from the eyelids to deep within the brain. It's more than poetic metaphor to say the eyes are an extension of the brain and central nervous system; it's an anatomical and functional fact.

An Inside Look at the Eye

Within the total physiology of the human body, the eyes are a prodigy of design and function. Anatomical estimates place the number of working parts of a single eye at one billion, including its 136 million photoreceptors, the rods and cones, which represent about 70 percent of our total sense receptors. Approximately 90 percent of the information most of us learn in a lifetime enters through the eyes.

The visual pathway begins with the eyeball itself, set within its bony socket called the orbit and bounded and protected by seven cranial bones. The bony eye sockets are lined with a cushion of fat that absorbs shocks and provides a lubricated surface for the eyes' constant motion. The smooth, rotational movements of the eyes are made possible by the cooperative work of three pairs of extrinsic muscles attached to each eye socket and the eyeball by elastic connective tissue.

Situated in the bony pits above each eye are the tear glands, whose secretions are essential for moistening the eye's surface. The automatic blinking of the eyelids keeps the eyes continuously lubricated, polished, and free of irritants. Blinking distributes a fluid containing oil and a powerful natural disinfectant across the eye's delicate outer transparent surface, the conjunctiva. The conjunctiva lines both the inner surface of the eyelids and the outer eyeball, which means that when you blink or shift your eyes the two lubricated conjunctiva surfaces glide smoothly over each other, protecting the vital inner parts of the eye from friction.

Underneath the conjunctiva's mucous membrane lie the eye's next two layers, the tough sclera and sensitive cornea. The sclera is the hard, opaque, wraparound protective layer, the "white of the eye." The sclera helps maintain the shape of the eye and is pliant enough to yield slightly to pressure. The cornea is a transparent, curved inner membrane made of bands of precisely aligned collagen nerve fibers. Its transparency is due mostly to the minimal presence of cells and blood vessels. The cornea slows incoming light and bends it, but without scattering or distortion, so that the retina, within the inner eye, can receive the intended visual image.

Immediately behind the cornea is a fluid-filled chamber called the aqueous humor. Its nutrient-rich, plasma-derived fluid, which is replenished every four hours, constantly nourishes the cornea and maintains its bulge, which is necessary for refraction.

Next along the visual pathway is the variously colored iris, named after the Greek goddess of the rainbow. The iris is a circular curtain of muscle that expands and contracts like a diaphragm around a central dark opening called the pupil. It does this according to the intensity of incoming light. The iris can change its size by as much as 17 times, from the size of a pinhead in glaring sunlight to that of a pencil eraser in darkness. By closing, the iris protects that delicate light receiver, the retina, further within the eye. When you see this sudden aperture change in someone's eye, it may seem that it's the black pupil changing, but it's actually the iris.

Were the iris completely rolled back like a curtain the full extent of the transparent lens would be revealed. Anatomically, the lens resembles an onion, comprised of numerous cellular layers added during life just like tree rings. The layers of the lens may number over 2,000, and as light passes through each micro-thin layer it undergoes a minute refraction. The lens of an 80-year-old is approximately 50 percent thicker than a 20-year-old's, and typically it has greatly reduced pliability and thus near-point focusing ability.

Ciliary muscles form a circular band around the eye. It is the contraction or relaxation of these muscles that automatically adjusts the shape or curvature of the lens to facilitate distance and near-point focusing. The maximum change in lens thickness is about 1/50th of an inch. The lens is round and convex when the point of light is distant, but when you need to see something in detail—up to the near-point limit of 6 inches—these muscles pull the lens into a concave, flatter shape.

Next on its long journey in to the retina, incoming light passes through the vitreous humor, a clear jellylike sac rich in protein fibers that lies behind the lens and occupies nearly two-thirds of the eye's volume. The vitreous humor is a transparent ball of jelly that maintains pressure within the eyeball. The vitreous humor also maintains the precise degree of light bending established earlier on the visual pathway by the lens. When dead blood cells drift through the clear vitreous gel, you experience them as "floaters."

After passing through the vitreous humor, light finally reaches the retina, layers of visual and nerve cells that cover about 65 percent of the eye's interior surface. Although the retina represents an estimated one-millionth of a person's total body weight, its nerve fibers account for 40 percent of all body nerve fibers entering the

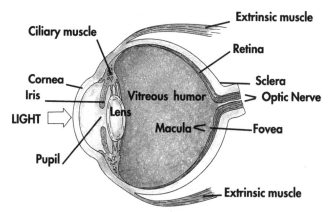

brain. The retina is the screen upon which the external image conveyed along the visual pathway from the outside world at last forms, though upside down. A "triumph of miniaturization," the sophisticated circuitry of the retina is capable of confounding even neurobiologists.

The retinal cells are packed closely to optimize visual acuity, and the retina is also exceedingly thin so that light can penetrate the outer layers of cells to reach the photoreceptors at the back of the retina. Here incoming light is transformed and coded into electrochemical signals to be sent down the optic nerve to the brain.

What accomplishes this remarkable translation of light energy into electrochemical signal in each eye are the millions of specialized photoreceptive cells called rods and cones. The more numerous rods operate in dim light and aid peripheral vision, while cones respond to bright light and provide detail and color. When magnified the cones look plump and bulbous, while the thin, straight, and densely packed rods resemble a rainforest thick with millions of waving tentacles. "If the whole population of the U. S. [then about 130 million] were made to stand on a postage stamp, they would represent the rods on a single retina," R.L. Gregory estimated in his book *Eye and Brain.*

The retinal screen has been likened to a painter's canvas, except that the artist paints from the back side of the canvas. That's because in terms of optical function the retina is inside out. The crucial light-sensitive cells are situated at the back of this multi-layered photonet, effectively facing away from the light. Incoming light must pass through blood vessels and a network of nerve cells before reaching the rods and cones.

At the retina's center there is a tiny dimple or pit called the fovea centralis, the only place in the retina that contains cones yet no rods. The fovea is directly aligned with the pupil, making it the eye's site of maximum visual acuity, detail, and overall clarity. The fovea is the only place in the retina where daylight has unobstructed access to the photoreceptors. The fovea's field of vision is minute—about 4 square inches at 8 feet—but it compensates for this size limitation through constant shifting of the eyes, another fundamental activity of seeing.

The distribution of rods and cones in the retina makes rapid adjustments to changing light conditions possible, a response called dark and light adaptation. When an eye adjusted to light is suddenly subjected to darkness, in the first minute of dark adaptation its sensitivity increases tenfold. After 40 minutes, it is fully dark-adapted, which means 30,000 times less light will still activate the retina.

Scientists have determined that sudden bright light bleaches the normally pink retina, which then gradually blushes red again. This bleaching-regeneration activity has been attributed to a visual pigment called rhodopsin, or "visual purple," found only in the rods. In the 1930s George Wald, a biologist at Columbia University, linked the presence of retinal vitamin A with the bleaching-regeneration cycle of visual purple. Wald found that the concentration of vitamin A (actually a chemical relative of carotene, the vitamin A pigment found in some plants and animals) in the retina increased as rhodopsin was bleached out from bright light and decreased as it regenerated and the retina flushed pink again. In other words, Wald discovered that vitamin A is a key factor in the chemistry of vision.

Seeing with the Whole Being

So here's how scientists outline the first steps in the process of normal vision. Light waves, reflected from an object in the environment, approach the eye. If the object is more than about 20 feet from the eye, the light waves move in parallel lines and are focused on the retina by the lens in its flattened, "at rest" condition. If light waves are coming from objects closer than 20 feet or so, the light enters the eye as divergent lines, requiring the lens of the eye to "accommodate" by forming a thicker, bulging shape to provide a sharp retinal focus. In other words, as light waves pass through the eye, they're bent, or refracted, and the degree of refraction determines whether a sharply focused image is cast on the retina.

The retina then converts the light input into electrical codes, and retinal nerve fibers carry the coded information through a densely packed transmission cable called the optic nerve to the brain. The two optic nerve cables each carry information from a single eye, but this dual visual message eventually converges to produce binocular vision. Here the visual pathway is complex, with data from each eye crossing over nerve pathways and finally being integrated and interpreted in the visual cortex, a folded sheet of neurons the size of a credit card located at the back of the brain. This primary sight-processing center is where "seeing" takes place. More correctly put, this is where eyesight becomes mind perception.

Somewhat like a television decoding visual information, the optic cortex converts the electrochemical messages sent from the retina's photoreceptors. The eyes haven't sent the brain any actual images, just electrical impulses, and these the brain must now decode and interpret. Here the brain changes sensory messages into conscious perceptions in acts of almost instantaneous recognition.

Current research indicates that visual signals are fed into three separate processing systems in the brain, for shape perception, color, and movement. Then the brain constructs a three-dimensional picture with depth and meaning.

All this happens so fast that it's far below the threshold of ordinary awareness. It takes less than one-tenth of a second for a retinal image to reach the visual cortex for analysis. And it happens very frequently, too. Each eye sends the brain about one billion messages per waking second, which is 430 times more data than the neighboring sense organ, the ear, transmits.

This brings us to the paradox of seeing and vision. Even though the visual pathway refracts and focuses incoming light through a complex, interdependent anatomical system, the essence of vision is cerebral. The mind interprets fresh visual data according to conceptual expectations, based on the person's life experience, culture, education, and other factors. It then projects the perceived image outwards again and we "see" it and respond accordingly.

Another way to express this is that vision is an active process of inference. The brain infers a three-dimensional image of the world, out of many possible configurations. On its own the incoming visual data is actually ambiguous.

So although we're born with sight, with open eyes ready to register the world, our brains must first learn how to see—and what to see. Plato once described vision as a process in which we send a ray of light out from the mind to collect images in the world. According to optometrists Arthur Seiderman and Steven Marcus, authors of 20/20 Is Not Enough, Plato was basically right. "The brain reaches out and imposes its individual meaning on the collection of messages it receives from the eyes," Seiderman and Marcus state. "Each of us creates his own visual world and it is unique."

"Seeing is not a separate isolated function," concurs Yale University vision development expert Arnold Gesell, M.D. "It's a process involving the entire human organism. The child sees with his whole being; it is profoundly integrated with the total action system of the child—his posture, his manual skills and coordination, his intelligence, and his personality."

The Essential Vison Functions

With this understanding of the anatomy of the eye and the science of vision, it's time to look at the major functional aspects of seeing: acuity, focusing, shifting, and fusion.

ACUITY. The norm for visual acuity is 20/20, based on the Snellen eye chart (see page 12). This series of boldface letters of different sizes, topped by a huge black E, was developed in 1862 by Hermann Snellen, a Dutch ophthalmologist. The Snellen chart is still universally used by optometrists as a primary test of acuity. Snellen's 20/20 standard means that at a distance of 20 feet you can sharply (or acutely) discern a ⅜-inch high letter in the third line of his chart. Snellen established this arbiter of visual normalcy on the basis of what an assistant of his with acute vision could see from 20 feet away.

According to one vision fitness estimate, if 20/20 represents 100 percent acuity, someone with 20/200 vision is making use of only 20 percent of the eye's visual acuity potential. You're legally blind if, with the best optical correction, your acuity is only 20/200.

Yet not all optometrists regard Snellen's acuity standards as absolute or inclusive. "The Snellen chart is a limited set of conditions," explains Stern. "It's high contrast, black letters on white, which isn't the way the world looks. The chart doesn't measure efficiency, visual style, or slight blurs. It's only a relative indicator that says if a person can read this in the office or classroom, when he's out in the real world, he'll be able to see most of the necessary things. For example, two people may both have 20/20 acuity but one may take twice as long to read the eye chart.

"I check acuity based on eye use and working distance—at 20 feet, then book distance, which is 13 to 16 inches, and also at 20 to 30 inches, which is where most people have their computer screens. We all work much closer up now than in Snellen's day."

Stern also warns against reducing vision to acuity only. She says, "Once I've ascertained there isn't an eye health problem behind the low acuity, I look at visual skills or abilities that relate to performance, such as eye movement, coordination, and convergence [the concurrent inward movement of the two eyes toward a near object]. There's much more to vision than the Snellen chart."

The Snellen Eye Chart

Based on a visual angle
of one minute

$\frac{20}{200}$	**E**	200 FT. / 61 m	**1**
$\frac{20}{100}$	**F P**	100 FT. / 30.5 m	**2**
$\frac{20}{70}$	**T O Z**	70 FT. / 21.3 m	**3**
$\frac{20}{50}$	**L P E D**	50 FT. / 15.2 m	**4**
$\frac{20}{40}$	**P E C F D**	40 FT. / 12.2 m	**5**
$\frac{20}{30}$	**E D F C Z P**	30 FT. / 9.14 m	**6**
$\frac{20}{25}$	**F E L O P Z D**	25 FT. / 7.62 m	**7**
$\frac{20}{20}$	**D E F P O T E C**	20 FT. / 6.10 m	**8**

12 **Seven Steps to Better Vision**

FOCUSING. This fundamental activity of vision is accomplished by the process of adjusting or accommodating lens shape for various distances. For an image to come into sharp focus on the retina, the diffuse outside light rays must be bent into a narrow, precise beam that is projected onto a tiny receptive area on the retina's surface. The cornea and aqueous and vitreous humors have an unchanging refractive power. The lens, by comparison, is flexible and can accommodate its physical curvature to complete the refraction.

SHIFTING. You experience your greatest clarity when you see through the fovea, that "tiny dot of perfect vision" within the center of the retina. The fovea sees only limited portions of the visual field with microscopic clarity at one time, but it compensates for this restriction by continually sweeping the visual field in rapid shifts. This shifting or "saccadic" movement happens about 70 times per second and has been likened to a gentle flapping motion like the flick of sails. When vision begins to deteriorate, the saccadic movements slow and become less frequent, vision blurs, and eventually habitual, excessive staring and eye strain result.

Foveal or central vision is prodigious. The continuous movement of the eyeball as it sweeps over the visual field point for point brings an object's full surface area into the concentrated photoreception of the cones. It's estimated that the unaided eyes, working together under the best viewing conditions, can distinguish 10 million colors.

FUSION. This refers to the eyes' ability to work together as a team, to converge the two images from each eye into one image, to see stereoscopically, and to have proper depth perception and peripheral vision. In short, fusion is the synchronous cooperation of both eyes in the act of whole brain perception.

Stern notes that the peripheral system involves spatial orientation and awareness, and is intimately connected with our motor system. She says, "Behavioral optometrists help people restore this ambient process because when it's impaired, it can have a profound effect on behavior. We work with children with learning-related vision disorders, adults with visual complaints from long hours at the computer, people with physical disabilities such as cerebral palsy or traumatic brain injury, and those with vision loss from accident or disease. These types of visual problems often go undetected but have a significant effect on a person's comfort, efficiency, and ability to achieve."

Common Vision Problems

For a variety of reasons, both physiological and psychological, the normal visual process doesn't always involve perfect acuity, focusing, shifting, and fusion. In fact few human eyes enjoy optically perfect refractive ability. Most people have some defect in curvature, density, position of eye structures, and variation in visual axis.

The widespread vision problem of nearsightedness comes about when the refractive power of the eyes is too strong, causing light waves to get focused slightly in front of the retina. This produces a blurred image of objects farther than 20 feet and in severe cases objects that are no farther away than 12 inches. Such nearsighted people clearly see only objects at near-point. Myopia is optometrically corrected by concave lenses that diverge light rays, pushing the focused image back onto the retina.

The opposite problem of farsightedness, or hyperopia, occurs when incoming light rays reach the retina before they've been adequately refracted by the cornea and lens. The result is a blurred, distorted visual picture for objects at near-point. Glasses with convex lenses are commonly prescribed for farsightedness because they converge light rays, restoring the intended focus of images to precisely on the retina.

How the Eye Focuses Light

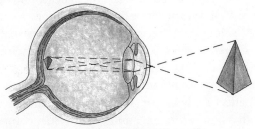

Normal eye function shows image reflected exactly on retina

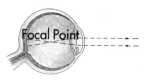

Nearsighted eye shows image reflected short of the retina

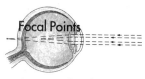

Farsighted eye shows image reflected behind the retina

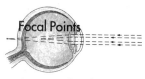

Astigmatic eye shows image reflected at more than one focal point

Presbyopia is the related condition in which the joint focusing system of lens and cornea diminishes during a person's later years. The eyes effectively freeze into an accommodation fixed on distant vision. Often known as "farsightedness of age" or "old man's eyes," it's so named because it typically affects people beginning around age 45, and particularly the elderly. Presbyopia is usually corrected by convex lenses used for reading and other near-point work. A presbyopic eye, however, is not necessarily farsighted. A presbyope can be nearsighted, farsighted, and astigmatic all at the same time, a complicated condition for which bifocals are usually the answer.

Astigmatism is another common refractive problem. Here the curvature of the cornea, and sometimes the lens, is defective. Rather than its natural spherical shape, the astigmatic cornea is elliptical, like the bowl of a spoon. The eyes thus refract light at differing angles and create various points of focus. The result is an inconsistently focused image in which some parts are clear but others are blurred and distorted.

These common vision problems are usually corrected by prescription glasses or contact lenses, but the eyes and visual system are sometimes subject to more serious functional and structural conditions, some of which are considered ophthalmological diseases. Crossed-eyes or strabismus is a functional problem in which one eye operates independently instead of working as a team with its mate. It may turn in, up, out, or down as it wanders around the eye socket. A related condition is lazy eye or amblyopia, which occurs when one eye progressively underachieves and stops functioning optimally. It's as if the brain tires of continuously integrating the divergent messages of both eyes and shuts down the weaker one.

Strabismus and amblyopia are fairly mild eye defects, but not so the "three great perils of sight": cataracts, glaucoma, and retinal diseases. These serious ophthalmological defects and pathologies are the proper concern of ophthalmologists.

A cataract is a cloudy, opaque, or filmy area formed by sediments in the lens. Vision with a lens cataract is like looking through a veil of flowing water. Cataracts develop gradually and can lead to loss of lens transparency, hazy or blurred vision, and blindness.

Glaucoma is a serious abnormality in which increasing pressure within the eye damages the optic nerve and impairs peripheral and central vision. It too can lead to blindness. The pressure within the eye builds up inappropriately because of inadequate drainage of the aqueous humor. As the fluid pressure builds up in the eyeball, it pushes the iris into the "angle" of the eye where the iris meets the cornea. As a result the iris completely blocks the eye's drainage system.

Retinal diseases include age-related macular degeneration (AMD), the leading cause of visual loss, particularly in people older than 65. This pathology takes two forms. In the first, a more prevalent condition called dry AMD, tiny yellowish deposits develop in the retina as the layer of cone photoreceptors lining the macula grows thinner. These changes produce dimmed or distorted vision. Wet or neovascular AMD, though less common, is a more drastic degenerative problem. Here new but abnormal blood vessels develop beneath the macula, leaking nutrient fluids and blood and causing the photoreceptor cells to sicken and die.

As a result straight lines become wavy and blank spots appear in the visual field.

Other retinal problems include tunnel vision or retinitis pigmentosa, a condition caused by degeneration of the retina's rods from genetic weakness or a lack of nourishment or stimulation. Vision narrows and peripheral and night vision deteriorate. Diabetic retinopathy is a degenerative condition that occurs in people with diabetes. Tiny superfluous blood vessels grow from the retina into the aqueous humor. When they eventually burst, bleed, and create scar tissue, blind spots appear and vision starts to deteriorate. A detached retina, in which the retina tears away from the sclera, often occurs after a sudden head blow. It's most prevalent among high myopes whose retinas are already considerably stretched thin because of elongation of the eyeball.

The Conventional Treatments

Conventional optometrists and ophthalmologists approach eye and vision problems with the same set of tools: corrective lenses, drugs, or surgical intervention, depending on the severity of the problem. The governing assumption is that functional, developmental, or genetic visual defects can be corrected only by mechanical intervention. Most of their patients don't expect anything else. Glasses are taken for granted, while surgery is becoming increasingly popular. A growing minority of doctors and patients, however, view some of today's expensive, high-tech medical procedures with skepticism.

For instance, one new and controversial surgical technique is photo-refractive keratectomy (PRK), which uses computer-controlled laser technology to make precise incisions on the cornea that correct errors in refraction. It evolved out of an earlier approach called radial keratotomy, developed by a Soviet ophthalmologist in 1975, in which a number of scalpel incisions are made in a bicycle-spoke pattern on the cornea to flatten it and thereby correct myopia.

According to one study of radial keratotomy done by the National Eye Institute, after the procedure 55 percent of the patients achieved nearly normal vision and didn't require corrective glasses, 28 percent remained nearsighted but with improvement, and 17 percent unpredictably became farsighted. On the whole about two-thirds of the recipients were able to eliminate their glasses, and after four years 76 percent of the patients had visual acuity of 20/40 or better without glasses. Even so, some eye doctors refer to the operation as "buccaneer surgery" and claim it is inadequately tested.

Ophthalmology has yet other surgical options available. In one procedure the outer layer of the cornea is removed, frozen, and reshaped on a computerized optical lathe. It's then sewn back onto the patient's cornea where it functions like a contact lens. The "living contact lens," another sophisticated eye surgery to reduce nearsightedness, involves suturing a portion of a donor's perfectly curved cornea onto the myopic cornea. The grafted tissue gradually integrates with the host corneal tissue to improve refraction.

Probably the most benign of medical approaches with the cornea is called orthokeratology, in which special contact lenses straighten the corneal curvature. This mechanical procedure—not unlike using orthodontic braces to straighten crooked teeth—can in some cases significantly reduce myopia in as short a period as 4-6 weeks.

As modern ophthalmology continues to develop increasingly advanced surgical interventions to improve eyesight or rescue vision from disease, few medical consumers stop to question whether it's all necessary. Isn't there something less physically invasive than photo-refractive keratectomy to improve nearsightedness? For that matter, are glasses unarguably, permanently necessary? Is one's natural vision irretrievably lost? If there is a practical holistic alternative to improve vision, what's it like and how does it work? These are questions anybody with glasses could ask. At the turn of the twentieth century, New York ophthalmologist William H. Bates, M.D., who was tired of his life with spectacles, did ask them. Along with a few other vision pioneers, he helped found what has become today's natural vision improvement movement.

One Hundred Years of Seeing Better Naturally

Advocates of natural vision improvement have been making a bold assault on vision orthodoxy for almost a century, though in various and sometimes competing forms. Three basic schools of vision improvement can be identified. The first was inspired by Bates and his book *Better Eyesight Without Glasses*, published in the early 1920s. Fans of Bates have included an assortment of writers, healers, and vision trainers, ranging from a prominent British novelist to one of the pioneer bodybuilders.

Around the turn of the century, roughly the same time Bates was developing his method, a second important wing of the vision improvement field germinated, this one made up of progressive optometrists. It has now developed into the field known as behavioral optometry.

Filling out the spectrum of vision therapists working today is an eclectic band of naturopaths, biofeedback practitioners, self-taught healers, and others advocating various holistic models of vision. These latter therapists offer practices, exercises, strategies, tools, and diets in various combinations and from a variety of sources, ranging from psycho-emotional work to yoga, chiropractic to hypnosis, herbs to massage.

Let's survey the development of these three somewhat overlapping branches of vision improvement, and then describe the seven-step approach that can help you to take advantage of the best and most practical suggestions from all of them.

The Bates Innovation

Based on his clinical experience, Bates said no, glasses aren't necessary in many cases and yes, refractive errors can easily be corrected by self-help exercises and attitudes. "I am well aware that I am controverting the practically undisputed teaching of ophthalmological science for the better part of a century," Bates confided. The medical profession had long sought a method for reversing the ravages civilization had wreaked upon the human eye, and now Bates claimed he had found one.

Bates argued his case on the basis of 40 years of professional practice. His ophthalmological credentials were among the best around. He had a large optometric practice that included "examining thousands of pairs of eyes" every year at the New York Eye and Ear Infirmary, along with regular surgery, teaching, consultations, and professional appointments at half a dozen of the city's prominent hospitals.

Though *Better Eyesight Without Glasses* wasn't published until Bates was in his early sixties, his work on vision improvement had been going on for years. Writing in a medical journal in 1891, Bates contended that nearsightedness could be eliminated through eye exercises. By the early years of the new century he had many satisfied patients who claimed to be seeing better without glasses. In 1912 he publicly opposed a plan to mass prescribe glasses for New York City schoolchildren. Shortly thereafter discomfited editors at the *Journal of the American Medical Association* received letters asking for details about Bates's "treatment for poor sight."

Bates said that it was his clinical observations that compelled him to proclaim "the uselessness of all the methods heretofore employed for the prevention and treatment of errors of refraction." That didn't mean the problem was unsolvable though, added Bates. It just required a different understanding of how the eye focuses light.

Modern ophthalmology's concept of how vision works was founded on the work of Hermann von Helmholtz, who in 1850 invented one of the profession's key tools, the ophthalmoscope. This tool allowed doctors to examine the interior of the eye. Early examinations led to one of ophthalmology's bedrock assumptions still in place today: that the lens changes its curvature by contraction of the ciliary muscles to accommodate near and far focusing.

Bates never accepted this view, however, believing that the mechanism of focusing is more complex.

The lens is not the sole factor in either focusing or in the correction of errors of refraction, Bates countered. Based on his clinical practice, he contended that it's the whole eyeball that changes shape according to the tension in the six extrinsic muscles that attach it to the orbit. It followed that deformations of the eyeball leading to refractive error and the need for corrective lenses are potentially temporary conditions. This concept of a temporary condition was perhaps the most controversial aspect of his findings, because it meant eye problems could be reversed and glasses thrown away. Conventional ophthalmologists were (and still are) committed to the view that corrective lenses are permanent necessities once a refraction problem has set in.

The root of most eye problems is mental tension and strain, said Bates. Fueling this continual strain are "wrong habits" of thought—trying to see with too much effort, or the empty stare of boredom. An eye operating under conditions of strain imposed by the mind loses its foveal seeing, so crucial to clear vision. When this goes, so does acuity. Only an eye that's completely at rest can experience perfect vision, said Bates. "The fact is that when the mind is at rest nothing can tire the eyes, and when the mind is under a strain nothing can rest them."

Bates also contended that glasses injure the eyes by forcing them into continually maintaining the same refractive error. The eye, whether normal, nearsighted, or farsighted, is far more dynamic, said Bates. It is subject to daily or even hourly shifts in refractive acuity. Bates called this the variability of refraction. He claimed to have never encountered an individual whose eyes maintained perfect sight for more than a few minutes, nor an individual with unchanging refractive errors. This of course makes the accurate prescribing of corrective lenses nearly impossible. "At their best it cannot be maintained that glasses are anything more than a very unsatisfactory substitute for normal vision," he concluded.

Bates proposed that relaxation, both mental and physical, is the key for the prevention and resolution of refractive errors. To facilitate relaxation, Bates promoted a series of disarmingly simple exercises, such as palming, blinking, and shifting (some of these are described in "Step One: Exercise the Eyes").

Bates substantiated his "revolutionary conclusions" by curing his own visual problem, "the maximum degree of presbyopia." Early in his career he couldn't read anything at close range without "an outfit of glasses" for various distances. It took him a year to justify his conviction and improve his accommodative range, using vision exercises developed from his studies. Fortified by his success, Bates believed he now had the practical credentials to encourage others to redress their vision deficits. "Fortunately for my patients, it has seldom taken me as long to relieve other people as it did to relieve myself," he said later.

Bates's work laid the foundation for a self-help, body/mind approach to vision improvement still thriving six decades after his death. One of his most literate advocates was the renowned British novelist Aldous Huxley, who used the Bates method to cure himself of a serious vision problem. In the early 1940s Huxley wrote *The Art of Seeing*, an eloquent and well-reasoned testimony that attempted to move the field forward by correlating the methods of visual re-education with the conclusions of modern psychology and critical philosophy. The book remains a popular work today.

Other early Bates fans included Bernarr Macfadden, the renowned bodybuilder and naturopath who wrote *Strengthening Your Eyes* in 1924, and Harold Peppard, D.O., an osteopath whose *Sight Without Glasses*, published in 1936, sold 500,000 copies. During the War years, the Bates method was hot. In Germany the Nazis officially adopted the Bates program, while in America young men rejected by the Army for poor eyesight tried eye exercises to improve their acuity. Thousands succeeded.

In the post-war decades, however, opposition from ophthalmologists increased and the Bates method lost its momentum in America. Until the late 1970s its practitioners were few and they worked in relative isolation. In the past decade the demand for Bates teachers has revived, though at present there is no national Bates organization. Many natural vision improvement teachers practicing today favor a blend of Bates's principles with techniques gleaned from other disciplines.

Progressive Optometry

The formative days of the second school of vision improvement, behavioral optometry, can be traced back to the vision therapy called orthoptics, popular in the late 19th century. It was concerned with what it called the straightening of the visual axis, or the eye's plane of vision. An early champion was the French ophthalmologist Emile Javal, who objected to the common practice of eye surgery for strabismus. To the outspoken Javal, such surgery was "the massacre of the eye muscles."

Rhythmic exercises would improve the eyes' ability to turn inward and focus on near-point objects, through training the nervous system to respond to acts of will, explained Claud Worth, M.D., an English ophthalmologist summarizing Javal's approach in 1903. David Wells, M.D., an ophthalmologist at Boston University Medical School, is credited with introducing orthoptics to the U.S. in 1912.

In the 1920s, A. M. Skeffington, a highly unconventional optometrist, advanced the field considerably and is now sometimes referred to as "the father of modern vision therapy." Skeffington "revolutionized clinical visual care, spurring the growth of what has become known as behavioral optometry," says Elliott B. Forrest, O.D., author of *Stress and Vision*. One of Skeffington's major contributions was to establish that the primary purpose of vision is to process information, which involves the entire visual system, from eye to brain.

In a radical departure from the conventional optometric view that regarded the eye as a mechanical camera and optical defects as genetic, Skeffington meticulously outlined a causal sequence showing how vision deteriorates. It all begins with excessive near-point work, which creates visual stress and tension, Skeffington said. This leads to a reduction and containment of visual space, a pulling in of the center of focus, and a restraint on accommodative movement. The next steps are over-convergence as a compensation and a constriction of the visual field. The result is a limitation of movement, learning, recall, and performance.

Further, said Skeffington, the standard Snellen chart and its 20/20 norm was seriously inadequate in its evaluation of visual performance. He pointed to numerous patients who had tested 20/20 yet had learning disabilities or were poor readers because of lack of eye teaming, poor focus, or convergence insufficiency.

Skeffington emphasized that one of the leading stressors of vision, particularly with children, is the prevalence of near-point work, in school and office. Skeffington considered excessive near-point work "an affront and insult" to the natural use of eyesight, branding it a principal factor in the onset of myopia. He reasoned, however, that if full, natural vision can be compromised by environmental factors like intense near-point demand, it could also be remedied and retrained, through a program of optometric visual therapy. Thus vision is essentially a learned skill, a view entirely at odds with ophthalmology's insistence that defective vision was structural and incurable.

Skeffington's bold work and his efforts to bring it to the attention of practicing optometrists nationwide led to the founding in 1928 of what is today the Optometric Extension Program Foundation in Santa Ana, Calif. The Foundation publishes the *Journal of Behavioral Optometry* and produces professional training courses, books, and consumer pamphlets. Its mission, according to current president James Cox, O.D., is "advancing human progress through education in behavioral vision care." The Foundation still uses the essence of an 18-point optometric examination that Skeffington developed as a comprehensive procedure to encompass his principles.

Today behavioral optometrists such as Cathy Stern number some 3,000 out of America's 24,000 licensed optometrists. They usually spend considerable time with each patient, taking a detailed personal history, inquiring about health problems and medical history, and discussing occupation and workplace conditions. Their principal intent, says Stern, is to relate visual problems to mind, body, and even behavior. "As a profession, we correct vision disorders that affect human learning, earning, and performance," she says.

"I'd love to be one of the people responsible for turning back the clock on visual deformation, eye problems, learning and perceptual difficulties, and the need for glasses," says behavioral optometrist Richard Kavner, co-author of *Total Vision*. Pointing out that modern American dentistry has helped to profoundly reduce tooth decay through education and prevention, Kavner says, "It's possible. But it requires education about how the eyes work best, lifestyle, nutrition, the proper use of glasses, how not to abuse the eyes, and the practice of visual training."

Vancouver behavioral optometrist and vision educator Robert-Michael Kaplan is the author of *Seeing Beyond 20/20* and a prominent innovator in the field. He's developed a 21-day vision fitness training program that includes vision games, exercises, nutrition, affirmations, and work with tools such as the eye patch. Kaplan's work has led him to conclude that an interdisciplinary approach to developing vision can produce "significant changes" in individuals' perception as measured by binocular optometric methods.

Behavioral optometrists stress the importance of, as Kavner put it, "treating the whole person and not just a pair of eyes," whether it's a child on the threshold of myopia or an adult with a 25-year history of high myopia. Visual training isn't something done to a patient, says Kavner. Rather, the therapist arranges the best conditions for the client to "permanently relearn how to see."

The Eclectic School

The selfcare, holistic view of health implies that clear vision can be reawakened by a variety of complementary measures. One of the pioneers of the third school of vision therapy was the outspoken British naturopath Harry Benjamin. "No one expects to cure defective vision by the aid of spectacles," Benjamin contended in his *Better Sight Without Glasses* in 1929. Glasses are a handicap, not an aid, to better vision and only make our visual disability worse, Benjamin claimed.

Like Bates, Benjamin spoke persuasively from experience—he said vision training had rescued him from "the valley of the shadow of blindness." When he was five, Benjamin was extremely nearsighted. The condition worsened such that by age 26 his optometrist gave him the strongest glasses for myopia then possible and dismissed his case as hopeless.

At that point Benjamin's brother read Bates's provocative book out loud to Benjamin, relating as well the successful results of a friend who had practiced the Bates method on his own, improving his sight tremendously. Benjamin knew "immediately and instinctively" that Bates's analysis of the cause of defective vision and its cure was right.

Benjamin "set about re-educating my eyes to see" and after only three weeks he could read without glasses, if slowly and painfully. By three years later, when he wrote his account, Benjamin had consolidated his vision gains and was able to read and write "quite well" without glasses. After Benjamin restored his vision, he became a Bates practitioner himself, expanding the basic approach to include dietary recommendations.

Benjamin's work inspired other naturopaths and alternative healers to explore the field of vision improvement. Like the natural foods movement and most holistic approaches to health and medicine, it bubbled along as an undercurrent of American society until streaming up to the surface in the 1960s. A flurry of vision improvement books incorporating ideas borrowed from nutrition, naturopathy, yoga, and psychology have appeared in the past two decades, such as Ann and Townsend Hoopes's *Eye Power*, Dr. Marilyn Rosanes-Berrett's *Do You Really Need Eyeglasses?*, Lisette Scholl's *Visionetics*, Christopher Markert's *Seeing Well Again Without Your Glasses*, and Janet Goodrich's *Natural Vision Improvement*.

One of the concepts that ties these writers and healers together is the whole person approach to vision therapy. According to Scholl, "I realized that in desiring to improve my vision, I was really desiring to grow as a person, to overcome basic reactions which had resulted in my closing down one of my sense organs, and to again see the world clearly, openly, holistically."

A second unifying concept is that all people are born with a natural ability to see clearly, and the brain never forgets how healthy vision works. Even those suffering from extreme nearsightedness or farsightedness can expect significant improvement. Kaplan reasons, "If the body can repair a wound on the skin, then why couldn't the eyes be trained to restore their natural way of seeing?" Martin Sussman, director of the Cambridge Institute for Better

Vision in Topsfield, Mass., calls clear vision "a capability that's always existed, just waiting to be reawakened." His self-help home practice program for vision improvement has reportedly aided some 24,000 people in restoring some degree of visual acuity.

Rejection of ophthalmological orthodoxy is a third common ingredient among natural vision improvement teachers. "The philosophy, education, and methods of natural vision education lie along a completely different path from that of orthodox eye practitioners," Goodrich maintains. She uses a variety of techniques including under-prescribed glasses, eye exercises, and psychologically-based drills. Like other doubters of the conventional vision wisdom, she's felt the wrath of skeptics and critics.

Controversy and Persecution

Vision improvement practitioners, whether followers of Bates, progressive optometry, or the eclectic school, have long been subject to ridicule or worse from the conventional ophthalmological and medical professions. As journalist Lawrence Galton observed, Bates had thrown a bombshell into the ophthalmological world and "it has been exploding in a chain reaction ever since." Even Bates did not escape the carnage: he was kicked out of the AMA for his heretical views on vision.

Margaret Darst Corbett, one of the first Bates practitioners, was the author of a number of vision improvement books and the founder of an eye-training school in California. She was arrested twice in the early 1940s for practicing optometry without a license. After she was acquitted both times, California eye doctors helped introduce a bill in the California state legislature that would have outlawed the advertising or use of any method of eye exercise or relaxation without an optometric or medical license. The de facto effect would have been to quash any teaching of the Bates method. Corbett and other Bates practitioners spoke out against the "eyeglass racket" and "medical monopoly," and the bill was defeated.

Clara Hackett, another Bates advocate and the founder of the American Association for Eye Training in Los Angeles, San Diego, and Seattle, was tried and acquitted in 1951 by a New York State grand jury for practicing vision therapy without a doctor's license. In 1974 Bates teacher Anna Kay of San Francisco was charged with 16 counts of breaking the law because of her vision therapy and an article she published on foot reflexology.

Probably the most virulent appraisal of Bates was issued in 1956 by Philip Pollack, M.D., in *The Truth About Eye Exercises*. He said that Bates's system was a pseudoscience "riddled with fallacies," his experiments were "demonstrably crude," he mistook testimonials for proof and rare anomalies for typical cases, his treatment methods were "totally without value," his ideas "sheer absurdity," and the whole system "a mental healing cult." Professional skeptic Martin Gardner is another vocal critic who has characterized Bates's work as "a fantastic compendium of wildly exaggerated case records, unwarranted inferences and anatomical ignorance."

Even today's behavioral optometrists criticize the Bates method as offering only "subjective improvement," in the words of Kavner. While not totally rejecting the Bates system, he insists that the results are often misleading. "What he said was accurate but not always for the reasons he gave…the methods were too imprecise, the claims too great, for it to be taken seriously."

Naturally, behavioral optometry also has its critics. The most vocal of these typically are the ophthalmologists, who contend that there's no proof that vision therapy accomplishes anything. Behavioral optometrists cite some 450 studies indicating clear benefits in about 80 percent of the cases. Critics such as George Beauchamp, M.D., a pediatric ophthalmologist with the Cleveland Clinic Foundation, rebut that the vision therapy studies are flawed and the facts of visual processing in the eye and brain don't theoretically support the therapies.

The American Academy of Ophthalmology and the American Academy of Pediatrics both reject the claims that vision therapy aids learning-disabled children or prevents juvenile delinquency. Part of the reason for the continuing controversy may be active resentment on the part of ophthalmologists and pediatricians at the way vision-training optometrists have encroached on their professional domain, suggest Ann and Townsend Hoopes. But more deeply it's the chasm between a structuralist and functionalist view of vision, say the Hoopeses.

The old school structuralists—the conventional ophthalmolo-gists—regard vision as a passive, mechanical, optical event. It is genetically pre-determined, independent of self-involvement, and correctable through lenses. The new school functionalists—the behavioral optometrists and vision therapists—see vision as an active, learned, and basically acquired and thus malleable process, correctable through visual training. "The functionalist believes that, through effective visual training including the appropriate use (for specific tasks) of stress-relieving lenses, the whole body/mind system will naturally reorganize itself in a more har-monious alignment," conclude the Hoopeses.

Holistic vision therapists also face their share of criticism and even harassment. "Education in natural vision training without the use of mechanical and optical devices is still beyond the imag-ination of some," confessed Goodrich. She says that during the 17 years she spent teaching vision improvement in Los Angeles, she was subjected to regular investigations by the State Board of Optometry. When in 1983 they sent Goodrich a letter stipulating that if she didn't clarify what her brochure meant by "visualization for better vision," the local district attorney would start an investi-gation, Goodrich had had enough. She obliged the state officials and then relocated to Australia, where she now teaches natural vision improvement with less governmental interference.

Seven Steps to Better Vision

The natural vision improvement field is clearly diverse. It presents what may be a bewildering array of options for the person inter-ested in learning how to see better without corrective lenses. From talking extensively to practitioners of all stripes as well as to their clients, and incorporating the most practical suggestions into my own quest for better vision, I developed the following seven-step program.

Step One: Exercise the eyes to enhance their ability to relax, focus, shift, work as a team, and visualize.

Step Two: Take advantage of the tools and techniques of behav-ioral optometry to optimize your ability to see with mind and body.

Step Three: Become aware of how hidden emotions and basic psychological attitudes may hinder vision, and practice some of the mental exercises that can help you overcome psycho-emotional obstacles to better vision.

Step Four: Learn how to free the body's energy channels and treat minor vision problems using natural remedies that range from acupressure to herbs.

Step Five: Become conscious of how movement, posture, and alignment of head, neck, and torso can affect vision, and use exercises and adjustments to correct patterns that can impair better vision.

Step Six: Feed your body and your eyes a diet—of foods, supplements, and light—for optimum visual health.

Step Seven: Learn and adopt the positive lifestyle and work habits necessary for the long-term health of the visual system.

Each of the next seven chapters is devoted to the information and practical suggestions necessary to implement these steps.

Part Two:
Seven Steps to Better Vision

Step One: Exercise the Eyes

Exercise the eyes to enhance their ability to relax, focus, shift, work as a team, and visualize.

Whether you call it ocular gymnastics, visual push-ups, or a natural method of vision rebuilding, there are numerous eye exercises to choose from to reclaim your natural vision. Although individual vision improvement teachers offer special exercises and tailored programs, in general the following exercises can help develop powers of relaxation, focusing, shifting, fusion, and visualization.

The exercises should be practiced without your glasses or contacts. As a variation, you can also try most of them with transition glasses, eye patch, or one of the other tools discussed in "Step Two: Work Out with the Behavioral Optometrists." It's important not to strain or attempt to overachieve in performing these simple drills. Remember to breathe calmly, deeply, and with awareness.

Relaxation Exercises

The following exercises relax the optic nerves, enhance blood circulation, and relieve muscular rigidity around and in the eyes.

PALMING. This is a method for resting the eyes in what Bates called "perfect blackness," a darkness free of all visual demands.

Rub your palms together briskly for about 20 seconds until you feel the sensations of heat and tingling. The rubbing energizes the palms. Cup the hands and place the palms over closed eyes, but without actually touching them or applying any pressure to them. Rest the fingers lightly on the forehead. Relax the mind by focusing attention on the breathing. Without straining or opening your eyes, see the blackness before you. One way to make the black more palpable is to imagine brilliant black suns in each palm expanding and enveloping the eyes in darkness. Practice palming for a few minutes or so several times a day while lying down on your back or sitting upright in a chair.

SUNNING. This exercise is best practiced when direct sunlight can strike the closed eyes at a diagonal—and that's usually before 10 a.m. or after 4 p.m.—and in short stretches of 2-5 minutes repeated a few times during the day. This exercise is not about getting a retina tan. It's about bathing the closed eyes in the nutrient of sunlight. Sunning stimulates and nourishes the retina indirectly, while relaxing the optic nerve. It also conditions the eyes to withstand greater amounts of light.

To practice sunning, sit comfortably, breathe with relaxation, close your eyes, and face the sun. Even when the sky is overcast, a great deal of sunlight is reflected off the clouds and will still be absorbed through the closed eyelids. Slowly move your head from left to right and back again, thereby continually exposing the surface area of your closed eyes to the healing radiation. Sunning can be interrupted after 3 minutes with a brief session of palming to further relax the eyes. The pronounced alteration from the light of sunning to the darkness of palming is palliative, making the pupils more flexible.

If direct sunlight isn't available, artificial light works well instead. For indoor sunning, use a low-intensity color-corrected incandescent light bulb or a full-spectrum fluorescent (see "Step Six: The Food and Light Nutrients" for a discussion of bulbs). You can work your way up to 60, 100, even 150 watts. Set the lights six feet away from your eyes with a reflector spotlight or screen around the bulbs.

Strobing is another variation on the eye sunbathing theme, suggested by Scholl. Sit down comfortably in a well-lit environment, preferably outdoors on a sunny day, and close your eyes. Hold your hands with fingers facing one another and slightly interlaced three inches in front of your face. Shuttle your hands up and down against each other to create a flashing effect on the closed eyes.

EYE BREATHING. John Selby, author of *The Visual Handbook*, devised this exercise to combine relaxation, mental imagery, breathing, and awareness of your eyes in a single practice. Sit comfortably in a chair, eyes closed, back straight, body relaxed.

Breathe calmly through the nose. Imagine that your eyes are inhaling and exhaling air as part of this same rhythmic cycle of the breath, as if your eyes have become lungs. Imagine, too, that energy, vitality, healing, and relaxation flow into your eyes with every inhalation, while what Selby calls "your own vitality and presence" flow back out into the world with your exhalation.

YAWNING. Deliberate, even exaggerated, yawning relaxes all the facial muscles, especially the jaw, while encouraging deeper, fuller breathing and better oxygenation. Behavioral optometrists and Bates correlated schoolroom boredom and blank staring with a rigidification of the eye muscles and a decline in central fixation, and a full yawn can help discourage these bad vision habits.

BROW ARCHING. Raising your brows relieves the heaviness and tension of the eyebrows, forehead, and upper eyelids that often impair easy movement of the eyes. Raise both eyebrows as if in complete surprise, and then lower them. Hold up the right eyebrow with your right hand and lower your left eyebrow with your left hand. Reverse the sequence.

BLINKING. You may assume blinking is an automatic, regular activity, but often people with refractive errors blink less than the average 20 times a minute. Reduced blinking leads to staring or squinting, both of which are harmful to the eyes because they halt shifting and foveal mobility. Deliberate blinking is simple: make dozens of delicate butterfly blinks for 10-20 seconds at a time, many times during the day, while gently sweeping the head from left to right. Frequent blinking momentarily rests the eyes, stretches the extrinsic eye muscles which might be chronically contracted, massages the eyeballs, and forces the pupils to continuously dilate and contract.

Focusing Exercises

The following focusing exercises can help strengthen the eyes' ability to quickly and effectively change their focus from near-point to far-point and then back again.

WATCHING THE BALL. Ball tossing, juggling, and watching sports such as tennis can improve visual mobility, accommodation, and focus because they enhance shifting. Constantly watch the ball, allowing the eyes to rapidly shift focus from near to far and back again. For example, take a tennis ball, toss it into the air, and track it visually without strain or holding the breath, blinking frequently. Alternatively, watch a live tennis or table tennis match, putting your complete but relaxed attention on the constant back and forth shuttling of the ball.

THUMB ZOOMING. This is an exercise that works with figure and ground focusing. Extend one arm straight out before you and point the thumb upwards, a little below eye level. Focus on this thumb, while breathing and blinking. Note the clear detail of your thumb framed against the general blur of everything surrounding it. Shift your focus to an object at least 10 feet behind your extended thumb. Expect that two thumbs will appear amidst the blurred background. Then zoom back and forth from thumb to background.

WHIPPING. Scholl says that she can't overemphasize the importance of this accommodation exercise, noting that it gets right at those spasmed ciliary muscles. Cup your right hand over your left eye. Extend your left arm out, fingers pointing upwards, palm facing inwards towards your face. Position your left palm as far to the left as you can still see with your right eye. Focus on your left palm with your right eye as you briskly move the palm in to within a few inches of your right eye. Whip the palm suddenly back to its initial extreme position on the left. This forces the right eye to nimbly shift focus. Whip a few times with this arrangement, then reverse. Block the right eye and whip the left eye with right palm movements.

TROMBONING. This is an effective focusing exercise suggested by Janet Goodrich. Take a standard table tennis paddle or a homemade paddle made of stiff cardboard and decorate it with colored stickers, dots, or images. Palm your left eye with your left hand and hold the paddle at arm's length in your right hand. Slide it in two-inch intervals toward your eyes as if it were a trombone shank. Trombone slowly at first, from the furthest stop into the position closest to your nose. Breathe calmly as your eyes accommodate to each new trombone stop. Next, trombone more briskly, adjusting the trombone stops from far to near, or play an eye tune as if you're the jazz master of the visionetics quartet.

EYE CHART WORK. This accommodative exercise cleverly makes use of the Snellen eye chart as a vision improvement aid. Bates praised the efficacy of even a half minute a day on the eye chart and urged schoolteachers to post one in every room. For the simplest use of the standard eye chart, place an enlarged copy on the wall significantly but not totally into your "blur zone." That means you can identify the chart without your glasses, but not very well. Read the smallest letters you can make out without squinting. If you can't make out any, move in a little closer. Let your eyes roam along the edge of the individual letters. Close your eyes and visualize the shape of each letter as big, black, and solid. Open your eyes again, palm the right eye, and read the chart with your left eye. Reverse.

Shifting Exercises

The following exercises discourage staring and help the eyes continually sweep the visual field in rapid shifts.

EDGING. This is a simple shifting exercise developed by Scholl. Sit comfortably, take off your glasses, and identify an object (a tree, a chair, a painting, a face) just beyond your range of clear seeing. Slowly and precisely trace the edges of the object, following its contours. Use your nose as a pointer as you edge the boundaries, moving your head naturally as you trace the form's shape. Then edge backwards. If you first edged clockwise, retrace the edge counterclockwise, allowing your fovea to shift in both directions.

To do a related exercise proposed by Meir Schneider, author of *Self-Healing: My Life and Vision*, take a page of printed material—this book, for example—turn it upside down and edge some letters. Blink constantly, breathe with attention, and don't struggle to read or decipher the reversed letters. That can wait until you flip the book right-side-up again and proceed to the next exercise.

NOSE DRAWING. As a variation on edging and shifting, draw the outline of objects as if a pencil or paintbrush were attached to your nose. Another variation is Goodrich's "General Electric" game, in which the nose pencil becomes an electricity-bestowing wand. First, hold your thumb upright before you at arm's length, then sketch it with your nose pencil. Next, imagine you turn on a hidden electric light bulb inside the thumb when your nose pencil touches it. Imagine that everything in your visual field has this latent light inside and you can switch on the bulbs with a nod of your nose pencil.

LONG STANDING SWING. Swinging is a gentle rocking motion that releases neck, shoulder, lower back, and spine tension, and exercises the whole body. At the same time, swinging makes the eyes more mobile, helps them shift more flexibly, increases blood circulation, and calms the nervous system. Swinging relaxes the eyes while encouraging them to make continuous, minute movements.

To do the long standing swing, stand with your feet parallel and 6-12 inches apart, arms hanging loosely. Face a window or even better stand outside in the sunlight. With your eyes facing straight ahead, sway from left to right, without pivoting the torso, by shifting your body weight from one foot to the other in a rhythmical fashion. Next, swing your body to the right, gently rotating your torso in that direction, with your weight on the right foot and the left heel raised slightly. Then swing to the left in the same way. Pivot your torso at the hips while turning your head in the direction of the swing. Keep your head level, attend to your breathing, and allow your eyes to remain entirely at rest, open and unfocused.

Look at the scene moving past you in the opposite direction of your swing, but don't pause to analyze, stare, or squint. You'll know an increase in foveal shifting is happening when it seems the room or scene slides past you in the opposite direction like railroad cars rolling across a landscape. This is a natural optical illusion produced by successful swinging. Try making 16 complete turns a minute, or about 60-100 swings per session.

SHORT SWING. Sit upright in a chair with an object such as a vase of flowers close at hand and another such as a wall painting more distant. While attending to your breathing, slowly rotate your head as if an elephant swinging its trunk, to the right and left, then back again. As before, don't actively focus on any objects before you. Swing your arms with your upper torso. Follow the short swing with neck rotations. In a slow, relaxed, and rhythmical manner, and with steady, aware breathing, draw an imaginary figure 8 in the air with your nose, then reverse the direction. The rotations smoothly move the head and neck in a wide, circular pattern.

THE NOTCHED CIRCLE. According to Selby, when you become aware of the shifts your eyes constantly make to apprehend an object, shifting happens with less tension. But first you must gain awareness of your chronic tension habits, which the following exercise suggested by Selby addresses.

Draw a large circle on a blank piece of white paper and then put 16 notches on the circle as if they were numbers on a clockface. Start with the first notch at the 12 o'clock position. For the duration of one breath look at that 12 o'clock notch. After a full, relaxed inhalation-exhalation cycle, move to the next notch and track your way around the circle.

As a variation draw another circle and put 12-16 prominent black dots or dense circles in random locations within. Place your attention on one dot, breathe regularly, and count to 20. Shift your perception randomly to another dot and repeat the breathing and counting. Then start with one dot, inhale for a count of 6 and exhale for another count of 6. After each inhalation-exhalation cycle, allow your eyes to randomly shift to another dot. Meanwhile continue the breathing, counting, and focusing.

Instead of black dots on white paper, sit in a room with reduced light, cover one eye, and use a flashlight held at arm's length to project horizontal, vertical, diagonal, and circular movements. Follow these with your single open eye while breathing calmly and deeply. Reverse eyes and repeat.

Fusion Exercises

Fusion exercises facilitate eye-teaming by deliberately moving both eyes in a systematic rotation. These exercises also stretch the eye muscles and enhance intraocular blood circulation.

THE EYE STRETCH. Sit comfortably and breathe consciously, blinking frequently. Close both eyes tightly, hold them shut for a few seconds, squeezing gently, then open them suddenly. Repeat this several times. On the exhale close both eyes tightly again. On the inhale, open them suddenly. Repeat this several times and relax completely. With your eyes open, look up with both eyes as far as possible without straining, then look down as far as possible. Keep your head straight and the neck and shoulders relaxed.

If you can do this without straining the eyes, look up when you inhale and down when you exhale, and then do 20 butterfly blinks. Look with both eyes as far to the right as possible and then to the left, doing this for ten cycles. Then do 20 butterfly blinks. Now look diagonally up to the right, down to the left, up to the left, and down to the right. Repeat this sequence ten times. For another variation, without moving your neck or head, roll your eyes to make circles around the periphery of your vision. Do this clockwise ten times and repeat counterclockwise for another ten cycles. As a final variation, practice the eye circles with your eyes closed.

BEADED-STRING FUSION. The fusion string exercise was originally conceived by a major figure in developmental optometry, Frederick Brock. It has many variations and names, but they all encourage individual eye images to fuse better, like twin color slides, to project a single perfectly focused image on the screen of the mind.

For this exercise, take a string or rope ten feet long, attach a bright bead or button (or tie a thick knot) every 8 inches, then affix the end of the beaded string to a wall or door. Sit comfortably in a chair, pull the string taut, and hold the end at your nose so that the entire beaded string extends horizontally from the wall. Breathing deeply, focus on the bead closest to your nose. The string will appear to split in two, crossing at the first bead to form an X. Slowly move your focus down the beaded string, pausing at each bead, until you reach the wall. Retrace your visual steps with each bead back to the one closest to your nose. Then jump from the nearest bead to the furthest and back again several times. Start at the second closest bead and shift focus suddenly to the furthest bead. Continue, starting at the third, fourth, and fifth, until all the beads have been focused on in reference to the furthest one. Practice this a number of times without straining. If eyestrain begins, stop, relax, blink, palm, and try again.

Next, repeat the bead sequence, this time passing quickly from each bead along the string to the wall, then back again to your nose. When you focus on the nose bead, suddenly shift your focus out to the last bead at the wall, then back again to the nose bead. Next, palm your right eye and repeat the movement down the fusion string using the left eye, palm the left eye, and repeat with the right eye open.

YARDSTICK FUSION. In this variation, substitute a yardstick ruler for the beaded fusion string. Hold the ruler horizontally such that one end is at your nose between both eyes, as if to measure the distance from your nose to something one yard in front of you. Focus on an object ten feet away in the room. Then move your eyes slowly down the yardstick's black notches, as if they were beads, starting at the notch closest to your nose. Continue until your focus reaches the wall. Again you're likely to experience the optical illusion of an X in the yardstick.

THUMB FUSION. Extend your arms straight out before you. Make a fist of each hand, point the thumbs upwards, and let the knuckles touch lightly. Focus on the space between the two thumbs and also at a point half the distance between them and your nose. Slightly cross your eyes. Without straining and while breathing smoothly, allow a third illusory thumb to appear between the two real ones. Maintain your perception of this ghost thumb for a minute, continue breathing, then look beyond your two thumbs to create a new phantom thumb in the distance. Shift your focus from the far imaginary third thumb to the closer imaginary thumb, then go back again. Stop when there are too many imaginary thumbs in the room.

FINGER FUSION. Here we give the thumbs a break. Hold your left hand six inches from your eyes and your right hand at full extension from your body. Extend the index fingers of each hand. Establish a third even more distant object for focus in this same line of vision as your two extended fingers. For one breath cycle, focus on the near finger. For the next, shift to the middle finger. Finally, shift to the distant object for another full breath cycle. Retrace your visual steps from far object to middle object to close. As before, do this in coordination with conscious breathing.

PENCIL FUSION. For this variation, substitute a pencil for your index finger. Extend your right arm parallel to the ground and hold the pencil vertically in your right hand. Stand about 10 feet from a wall to which you've attached a standard index card. Look at the card on the wall. You'll probably find the pencil doubles in your perception. Shift your focus to the pencil and notice how the wall card doubles while the two pencils return to one. Repeat this several times. Move the pencil closer to your eyes in one-inch increments until it's about 3 inches from your nose. With each incremental move, check the wall card again.

THE SWINGING BALL. This comprehensive exercise activates and integrates the two hemispheres of the brain to produce what Kaplan, its originator, calls "synchronous whole-brain perceptions." Attach a tennis ball by a string to the ceiling such that it hangs about 16 inches from your eyes and directly overhead as you lie on a bed, couch, or the floor. First, observe the ball as a clear figure framed by a blurry background. Use the hanging ball to practice thumb zooming as described above. Next, push the ball so it swings back and forth from your feet to your head. Track its movement with your eyes, staying aware of the rise and fall of your breathing. Start the ball swinging from left to right. Again, track its motion without straining or moving your head. When the ball crosses the midline of your vision, between your eyes, you may experience the hemispheric switching of perception in your brain. Practice ball swinging for 20-50 breaths.

Visualization and Imagination

"Perfect memory of any object increases mental relaxation which results in a relaxation of the eyes and both together result in better vision," Bates explained. He was reminding us that memory facilitates vision. Visualization develops inner memory, and this is essential to vision because you perceive familiar objects more easily and clearly than unfamiliar ones. The aberrations of myopia are illusory, Bates argued, and are correctable. "A perfect imagination not only corrects the false interpretation of the retinal image but corrects the error of refraction," he said.

FLASHING. Glance at an object or scene, close your eyes momentarily, and remember what you've just seen. Flashing is like the perceptual reverse of blinking—you blink in quick imprints while your eyes are open. These rapid, relaxed flashes of perception enable you to see with detachment, free you from habitual visual anxiety, and produce a sharper, more acutely detailed image.

The strategy of the following memory and imagination exercises is that while the retina records a visual pattern, it's the brain that interprets this pattern, turning it into something meaningful. Memory helps the whole process. It gives the brain clues and practice in interpretation. To see with high visual acuity, you require a precise mental concept of what it is. Although it's paradoxical, it seems the eyes see what the mind expects them to see and the mind sees it before the eyes do.

THE BLACK DOT. Using black ink draw a solid dot the size of a freckle on white paper, or draw the dot next to a large letter on the eye chart. Without staring or straining, and while breathing regularly and deeply, examine this black dot until its blackness registers completely. Retain this image, close your eyes, and remember the same black dot. Bring that black dot perfectly before your inner attention. Next, open your eyes and examine an eye chart letter while retaining the mental picture of the black dot. Superimpose the dot over the large E until they merge. Close your eyes and imagine the black dot without having actually seen it first on the chart. Open your eyes, superimpose the mental picture of the dot again on that same E. Next, substitute another letter for the black dot and repeat the sequence. Then substitute simple objects in your environment for the black dot.

THE O SHUTTLE. This dynamic visualization was suggested by Corbett. Close your eyes and imagine a large, black, round letter O. As if the O were a clockface, put a large bulging black dot at the 12 and 6 o'clock positions. Retrieve your nose pencil. As if you were seeing this O on a large imaginary chart before you, track its outline back and forth between the 6 o'clock and 12 o'clock dots with your nose pencil. Slightly move your head as your inner eyes shuttle across the clockface O. Next, put a similar black bulging dot at the 9 and 3 o'clock positions on the O, and repeat the imaginary shuttling. Finally, shuttle back and forth between the 12 o'clock and 6 o'clock dots.

DOMINO MEMORY. For this memory training exercise, developed by Rosanes-Berrett, you need 14 standard dominoes with white dots against a black background. Stand the dominoes an inch apart at face level, left to right, the white dots facing you. Position yourself on the edge of your blur zone. Close your eyes, relax, and breathe deeply. Open your eyes and lightly examine the contours of the domino farthest to your left. Imagine that you are seeing from the back of your brain, from the optic cortex, the seat of visual processing. Close your eyes and then visualize this same domino you were just examining, intensifying its image until it grows precise and sharp. Open your eyes and repeat this style of domino-looking six times using the same domino. Next, shift your attention to the neighboring domino and repeat the sequence of outer gazing followed by inner visualizing. Do all twelve dominoes. As a variation use playing cards with numbers taped to the wall in a horizontal line, or a calendar whose large numbers in blocks will replace the rectangular dominoes.

COLORING THE EYES. This powerful color visualization was developed by Martin Sussman. It involves moving individual healing colors through the visual routing system in coordination with the breathing cycle and a mental imaging of the general anatomy of the eyes, brain, and optic nerve.

Sit comfortably, close your eyes, and relax into a natural breathing cycle. Visualize that your left eye is filled with bright yellow light, as if the sun were glowing there. Slowly move this yellow sunlight back up the optic nerve into the visual cortex of your brain, then into the left occipital lobe, to the right occipital lobe, to the right optic nerve, then out through the right retina, the lens, cornea, and sclera.

Putting Together a Personal Exercise Program

If you're looking for the easiest, quickest way to practice these exercises, try working them into some aspect of your daily routine. For instance, I live on a lake and canoe each day. The canoe has become my optometrist's office. Out on the lake, I carefully stow my glasses in my front pocket and start by palming and sunning my eyes. I yawn and do butterfly blinks and a few rounds of eye stretches. I look at my two hands on the canoe paddle, shift my sight to the front end of the canoe, then out to the shore and back again. I turn on light bulbs inside each leaf of the trees on the shore. Across the cove I edge the outlines of the oak, maple, and birch trees against the clear blue sky. I strap on my nose paintbrush and paint. Next, I may edge the green light cones reflected by the trees in the still water.

Other people who have used eye exercises to improve their vision have developed routines that they do while walking in the woods or sitting at a desk. They may take five minutes to perform the exercises once or more each day, or devote half an hour. What's most important is finding out what works best for you and how much time you can spend, and then approaching the exercises not as work or drudgery but as a chance to play with your vision and improve it at the same time.

Step Two:
Work Out with the Behavioral Optometrists

Take advantage of the tools and techniques of behavioral optometry to optimize your ability to see with mind and body.

In the mid-1970s Ann Hoopes was 42 going on 50. She was plagued by a long list of medical problems, including the after-effects of a hysterectomy, menstrual irregularities, serum hepatitis, spastic stomach, chronic headaches, and postural imbalances. She also had vision problems, including 20/100 nearsightedness and astigmatism. It was "a near-total collapse of my health," she confesses, that left her depressed and frustrated.

These problems should not be insurmountable, however, she was told when she first visited a doctor practicing the specialty of behavioral optometry. He contended that her health problems were due largely to her defective vision. He prescribed several "therapeutic lenses," glasses with a lower prescriptive power than would give her 20/20 acuity. He also started her on a series of eye-training exercises and taught her how to use a variety of vision-enhancing tools. The objective was to dislodge Hoopes from her unhealthy visual/postural habits and to help her to develop new patterns that reflected harmonious eye/mind/body relationships.

Hoopes noticed positive changes even the first week. Twice over the next two years she experienced the crucial "transition," a moment in which she perceived her shoulder muscles, blood vessels, and neck bones literally shifting and realigning, bringing her posture into new alignment with her eyes. The momentary discomfort brought rich rewards.

"When I went to eye-training class the following day, I looked out the window and found the streetlights actually popped out at me." In mid-life she was "finally discovering the third dimension." Within three years nearly all of her physical symptoms and difficulties had cleared up, her vision was an entirely reborn experience, and she felt her prospects for "even better bodily health and further growth in visual perception and mental efficiency" were highly promising. The new visual training available from behavioral optometry, she said, "offers the prospect of extraordinary benefit to those who are motivated to undertake it. Total performance is the payoff."

Beyond the Optical Theory of Vision

Ann Hoopes's remarkable success with behavioral optometry sets the discipline and its principles in dramatic relief. Difficulties or obstructions in the processing of visual information—visual stress, in short—not only impair clear seeing but often produce diverse, seemingly unconnected problems in behavior, social adjustment, learning, work, and intellectual efficiency. Health problems involving posture, insomnia, digestion, and energy level are also common.

With this causal relationship in mind, the behavioral optometrist sets out to optimize the functioning of a variety of visual skills. In addition to the commonly recognized ones of acuity, focus, shifting, and fusion, they work on depth perception, peripheral vision, maintaining attention, and visualization. Behavioral optometrists also consider less conspicuous visual processing problems not always associated with underachieving eyesight, such as visual-verbal match, directionality in space, figure-ground perception, visual form perception, and visual-motor coordination.

The idea behind behavioral optometry is that better eyesight results not only from improving acuity or Snellen rating, but through correcting "warps," imbalances, or developmental lags at any point in the visual pathway. Vision isn't merely seeing with the eyes or brain. It's the whole person receiving and processing visual information.

In this view, a purely optical theory of vision is altogether inadequate. The brain, the mind, the person, the body's physiology and orientation in time and space are all actively involved in the process of seeing, or compromised when the process is skewed. Vision is the dominant motor-sensory system. It's the "master coordinator, affecting and affected by every other component of the body/mind system," explain the Hoopeses in *Eye Power*.

Clearly vision involves much more than the ease of reading big black letters on a chart. It implicates all your vision-based behavior—and that doesn't leave much out. Hence the name of the specialty. "It follows that you cannot improve your eyesight, except very temporarily, without also improving your overall performance," according to the Hoopeses.

The therapeutic lens is a hallmark of behavioral optometry, which commonly prescribes them for remedial, developmental, and preventive purposes, but it's a discipline that embraces a lot more than the correct use of glasses. Reduced-strength prescription lenses are one of a number of innovative tools, including other types of specialized glasses, the common eyepatch, biofeedback machines, and even the trampoline, now being used by progressive optometrists and natural vision trainers. In their offices, they may also offer such tools as rotary devices (moving disks with pictures) and balance boards or beams.

Beyond these physical tools, behavioral optometrists and others are concerned about the correct use of vision itself. Vision therapy, state Seiderman and Marcus, isn't so much about what happens in front of the retina, where refractive errors in seeing are attributed to changes in the shape of the eyeball. It's about what happens behind the retina, "in the interaction between brain and eyes—the world of vision. Vision therapy is a form of neurophysiological treatment for disorders or dysfunctions, not disease. Since the causes of all visual disorders lie in the messages sent by the brain to the eye, that is also where the cure takes place." We're born with sight, but vision is learned, emphasize Seiderman and Marcus. They attempt to teach the brain to "send the right messages to the body....The instruments we use are designed to help create situations in which the brain finds it natural to give those correct instructions."

Using Therapeutic Lenses

Students of progressive optometrist Robert-Michael Kaplan typically carry an assortment of differently prescribed glasses in their purses or satchels. In the course of a day they may wear them all, changing their refraction according to their activity and which aspect of their brain chemistry they want to access, says Kaplan.

"This opens up a whole new understanding of lens prescription," claims Kaplan. "The old system of prescribing glasses only creates addictions to refractive compensations. When you're wearing therapeutic lenses, you're continually in therapy all day, engraving new habits of perception."

Natural vision trainers contend that when a conventional optometrist writes a lens prescription to restore a patient's acuity to approximately 20/20, the ability of the eyes to adjust their focus from far-point to near-point essentially gets frozen at that one prescriptive level. The eyes are given no incentive to improve. In fact, standard prescription lenses prevent it.

"Glasses are often called corrective lenses, but they don't really correct the problem," says Cathy Stern. "If you take your glasses off, you're just as nearsighted today as when you got them. I call them compensating lenses because they compensate for the change—usually the reduction—in sight. Eyeglasses treat the symptom but not the cause."

As she prepared a reduced-prescription lens for me, Stern continued, "It's like never having exercised some important muscles for years. These weaker lenses will force your eye muscles to stretch after a long period of relative inactivity. Your glasses have done all their work for years."

Under-prescription is a prominent tool in trade for behavioral optometrists like Stern and Kaplan. For some myopes and hyperopes willing to try a different approach, it can mark the transitional stage from requiring glasses to being occasionally or even permanently free of the need for them. It is based on two startling concepts. One, that glasses and contact lenses might be a type of visual crutch. And two, that there are ways to actually improve one's eyesight, the controversial notion that figures prominently in holistic vision programs.

Referring to my nearsightedness, Stern says, "There might be an interim period when your eyes haven't gotten stronger yet and you can't tolerate that distance blur." It takes about two months for the body to come into balance with the kind of major visual change an under-prescription like this affects. "Just wear your old glasses for distance seeing or driving," Stern says. "Gradually we can stabilize your prescription at a lower level than where it's been for years."

Varying prescriptive lenses offer "a noninvasive way to control information entering the visual system," concur Seiderman and Marcus.

Kaplan himself doesn't wear any glasses today, but years ago he had such major visual problems as double vision, dyslexia, and learning disability. Bifocals and special prisms were the only corrective means optometry offered him so he resolved to try holistic remedies. "I began eye exercises to reprogram my brain and eyes to see single," he says. When prescribed therapeutically, glasses can actually perform their intended function to correct, not compensate, refractive error. "The goal is that you wean yourself down the scale to a point where you are, from a whole person point of view, physically and psychologically, ready to see clearly again."

Kaplan founded this conclusion on several key observations. First, about 95 percent of the time optometrists prescribe full-strength glasses to produce 20/20 refraction to match what's considered to be the norm of visual acuity. "But in my research on stress and two-eyedness, I have found that in 75 percent of cases, full-strength lens prescriptions for nearsightedness and astigmatism produce distress—unmanageable stress—related to how patients use their two eyes together." Second, most optometrists determine the lens prescription by testing each eye separately. They assume that a "single-eye tested" prescription will work satisfactorily in "two-eyed seeing," that through eye-teaming the separate lens compensations will work together and average out.

Kaplan's clinical research convinced him that single-eye tested prescriptions were too strong and probably lowered a client's vision fitness. Kaplan's approach has been to test both eyes while open and to prescribe reduced strength lenses. Through experimentation, he found that the reduction level that still encouraged optimum vision fitness was 84 percent, or correction to about 20/40. This gives just the right amount of blur—the eyes can manage it but they're challenged to improve. If we liken the eyes to an injured arm bound in a tight splint, wearing weakened glasses loosens the splint so the arm is flexible while still supported. "This means that by introducing some vision fitness exercises into your daily routine, you can train your brain, eyes, and muscles to make up the 16 percent difference. After a period of time you will be seeing 20/20 through this same vision fitness prescription. The stronger glasses keep us locked into one visual reality. It brings more stress and isn't a healthy state. A reduced prescription with a therapeutic design is a natural anti-stressing, healing program," Kaplan says.

Not only does Kaplan deliberately challenge the eyes to see better through under-prescribing the compensation, but he contends that one prescription can never meet the range of our visual demands. Following Bates's indication, Kaplan appreciates that an individual's refractive error is dynamic, not static, and fluctuates considerably across the Snellen chart on a daily or even hourly basis. And as Stern pointed out, your vision naturally accommodates to the demands of the specific activity, whether it's nearpoint or distant-point—and so should your glasses. But that's technically impossible because conventional prescriptions typically lock the eyes into one unvarying correction. If you have a refractive deficit then you best serve your eyes by having a different prescription for each kind of activity. It's a way of achieving accommodative flexibility through having a lot of different lenses on hand.

Kaplan therapeutically accentuates the blur through the precise use of lens strength, whether it's an under-correction for myopia or an overcorrection for astigmatism. For instance, he said, for someone with vision like mine, "I would 'blur back' your dominant eye by under-correction. Then you have to look more through the weaker eye. The effect is similar to wearing an eye patch."

The complete elimination of our glasses isn't necessarily the mark of success, Kaplan reminds us. You can heal your vision problems and still wear glasses because where you start compared to where you finish can be considerable. "We start off with our vision restricted so we use the glasses as compensations," he says.

"When we use the lenses intelligently, our eyes are freed for vision. What we're changing is inner vision in the mind, using our eyes as steering wheels. This is the psychological aspect of perception, how vision is driven as a projection of the mind. I look at how we can modify the psychology of perception and behavior through the application of therapeutic lenses in conjunction with a vision improvement program."

From Pinholes to Prisms

Behavioral optometrists also employ a number of special glasses and lenses that alter how the eyes transmit light input to the brain, and thus how you see.

PINHOLE GLASSES. Pinhole glasses, first developed in Germany in 1896, are now available in a number of patent variations on this basic design principle. Pinhole glasses are regular eyeglass frames equipped not with clear glass or plastic lenses but rather thin lenses of black plastic honeycombed with approximately 170 tiny round holes. The holes break up the incoming light, and thus the visual burden, for each eye, by allowing only parallel rays of light to enter the eyes. This enables the retina to focus easily while eye muscles relax.

The narrow rays of light on the retina also create much smaller blur circles than result from the broad sheets of light that normally enter a nearsighted person's eyes. You can demonstrate this action by punching a tiny hole in a piece of paper, or forming a loose fist. Close one eye and put the hole in the paper, or your fist with a tiny opening in it, to the open eye to peer through. If you're nearsighted, you'll see distant objects with surprising clarity using this makeshift one-pinhole telescope. Pinhole glasses work similarly to allow the eyes to relax and to see more clearly.

Pinhole advocates claim that some degree of increased visual acuity is almost always the case regardless of one's initial error of refraction. Pinhole glasses can be worn initially for 10-15 minutes, then up to an hour a day, during eye exercises or general activities (not driving or night vision) that pose only a modest visual demand. After a few minutes of seeing the world through separate pinholes, the tiny apertures in the central area of the glasses seem to merge into one opening, while the peripheral pinholes keep the visual field perforated and outlined in black.

ANAGLYPH GLASSES. With one green lens and one red, anaglyph glasses work along a somewhat similar principle. The idea is to deliberately segregate the information from the eyes by subjecting each to a different color. One eye sees the red, the other sees green, and the brain has to integrate information from both eyes to "see" a single target in three dimensions.

Marcus cites a recent case from his own clinical practice. A man in his late twenties came to him complaining of headaches, eyestrain, fatigue, and loss of efficiency. The patient spent eight hours a day at a desk including five hours working at a computer terminal. He already wore glasses, and his conventional optometrist said no change in prescription was necessary so there was nothing else to offer for help. "Our view was that this man had convergence insufficiency, which is the single most common binocular dysfunction," comments Marcus. This is an inability to sustain coordination between the eyes while working at near-point, such as using a computer terminal. The two eyes produce conflicting images instead of working together as a team to converge an image into a single focus.

Among the tools Marcus used were anaglyph glasses, similar to the ones used for 3-D movies. While wearing the anaglyphs, the patient focuses on two clear sheets of plastic, each of which bears an inscribed circle. The sheets of plastic are backlit and positioned so that the circles are next to each other but not overlapping. The patient views this image at varying distances, starting at 18 inches and progressing to about 20 feet. Eventually the brain fuses the red information from one eye and the green from the other to produce an image of a third circle between the two inscribed on plastic. Marcus had the patient work with anaglyphs about 10 minutes a day to get immediate feedback on his progress in seeing a single three-dimensional color target.

The results of this simple test indicated whether one eye shuts down in the attempt to achieve convergence and depth perception. Wearing these glasses also promotes three-dimensional seeing and encourages the brain to integrate information from both eyes to see a single object in the environment.

POLAROID GLASSES. Polaroids, like the anaglyphs, separate light in a way that encourages the brain to rely on both eyes for a converged image. Resembling dark sunglasses, Polaroid lenses have specially laminated sheets embedded with tiny crystals that polarize light. That is, the field of the light wave is confined to one plane or one direction. Typically with Polaroid glasses, the axis of polarization for one lens is 45° while the other is 135°. The effect is to have light enter the right eye in a different direction than the light that enters the left. Using the same backlit, clear plastic sheets with circles, the patient does exercises that stimulate better depth perception.

PRISMS. Special prisms can be incorporated into everyday lenses or, in stronger versions, used with special therapeutic lenses during office visits to your behavioral optometrist. A "directive prism" is worn continuously to re-arrange space so one's perception is reorganized. It works at an unconscious level in which corrections happen without one being consciously aware of them. A "disruptive prism" causes an easily recognized change in visual input. The effect is to stimulate the eyes to move in and out of seeing in tandem or alternately stimulate and relax the accommodative system.

Anaglyphs, Polaroids, and prisms are routinely prescribed by behavioral optometrists according to the individual optical conditions of patients and shouldn't be used without their professional consultation. Also, although behavioral optometrists are likely to make this clear, it's important to emphasize that you shouldn't wear under-prescribed lenses, pinholes, anaglyphs, Polaroids, or prisms for activities such as driving or operating power tools. These specialized tools of behavioral optometry should be used at home during activities with reduced visual demand, such as reading or walking.

Patch Power

The eye patch is a popular tool commonly available through vision improvement programs and catalogs. It's also simple to make at home. The patching idea is to temporarily block off the dominant eye, encouraging the weaker eye to do all the seeing. Patients wear the patch initially for brief periods of 10-15 minutes, building up to an hour or more. The patch should not be used for strenuous or near-point visual work, such as reading or driving, but rather for activities such as walking, gardening, or doing housework.

There are several variations to the patch. Place translucent tape over the lens of your glasses for the dominant eye, then wear them as a spectacle patch. The translucent tape allows light to pass through to the eye but not distinct images. This stimulates the photoreceptors of the weaker eye to "wake up" and start seeing again. The two-eyed patch, suggested by Kaplan, encourages peripheral vision. Cut a strip of cardboard into a 3-inch by 1-inch section, with a triangular section removed from the bottom middle to accommodate the bridge of the nose. Secure it gently to your forehead with a strip of masking tape and do low-visual-demand activities or eye exercises.

Covering one eye at a time with a black patch can have both physical and psychological effects on vision. Let's say a person's right eye is dominant. Psychologically, this corresponds to perceptions associated with the left brain's rational, analytical correlates. When the dominant right eye is blurred, the weaker left eye is challenged to see more, to contribute more to the vision process. The left eye corresponds to perceptions associated with the right brain, the intuitive and visual hemisphere. The overcorrection of the right eye (through accentuating its astigmatic blur) compels the left eye into activity, and may help to access those right-brain qualities of creativity, imagination, and intuition. "You're in your feelings more," comments Kaplan. "This is useful for myopes who tend to keep their emotions tightly controlled and stay in their minds, in their left brains, all the time."

Biofeeding for Vision Training

Using biofeedback instruments, behavioral optometrists have stopped or reversed myopia in thousands of people of all ages. One of the most effective such devices, says Steven Marcus, is a relatively new high-tech machine known as the Accommotrac.

Marcus is one of about 200 O.D.s in America with one. The Accommotrac "holds out hope to almost all kinds of myopes," says Marcus.

Back in 1981 Joseph Trachtman, O.D., a behavioral optometrist practicing in Brooklyn Heights, N.Y., completed seven years of research and development and presented his Accommotrac Vision Trainer to the optometric world. Trachtman coupled the sensitive interactive nature of biofeedback with the accommodative principle of optometry so that patients could learn to actively control the crucial act of shifting focus, thereby overriding the automatic function which in myopes is chronic tensing and contraction. The concept is that if a person can consciously keep the eye muscles relaxed while focusing, acuity will substantially improve.

Through interaction with the Accommotrac and monitoring its direct feedback, the patient discovers a voluntary action—whether it's imagining a landscape or sound or getting a muscle to relax—that will produce the involuntary action of the ciliary. The feedback reveals the unique physical pathway by which a person can relax the ciliary muscles and see better by his or her own efforts.

The Accommotrac works by having the patient gaze through an eyepiece into a field of white light, one eye at a time. The eye reflects back this light and the Accommotrac instantly determines the degree of tension or relaxation of the ciliary muscles of each eye. It is sensitive enough to pick up minute changes at the rate of 40 per second. The Accommotrac then translates these miniscule fluctuations into sounds and a numerical graph. The therapist asks the patient to make the sound change in a way that reflects increases in relaxation of the eye muscles. The Accommotrac feeds back to the patient information on how successful he or she is. The patient's goal, explains Marcus, "is to find a voluntary action—imagining a sound or landscape, or relaxing a voluntary muscle—that will trigger the involuntary response of the ciliary."

On the basis of various studies and his own clinical work with the Accommotrac since 1987, Marcus contends that "the great majority of nearsighted people can expect substantial improvement." A 1985 survey of 16 nearsighted people, aged 9-37, culled from New Jersey optometrists using the Accommotrac, showed that all the patients were less nearsighted after treatment. For instance, a 20/30 patient improved to 20/20, while a 20/400 one radically reduced her myopia to 20/100. In Trachtman's own study of 84 patients, the initial acuity ratings ranged from 20/20 to 20/1000. After eight sessions on the Accommotrac, acuity ranged from 20/15 to 20/100. *Omni* gave the subject national attention in 1985 when it reported the case of Robert Mucci, a man with 20/400 myopia who desired to become a New York City firefighter—that is, if he could lower his nearsightedness to 20/40. He did, after 20 sessions with Trachtman. "Biofeedback has provided vision therapy with a powerful new tool," observes Marcus.

Working Out in the Eye Gym

If people could only practice vision therapy as a preventive health care measure in early childhood, when problems first begin developing, then they'd see a radical reduction in later visual dysfunction. That's the basic drift in the thinking of many concerned behavioral optometrists, including Raymond Gottlieb, O.D., Ph.D., who's doing something practical about it. Back in 1970 Gottlieb improved his myopia from 20/60 to 20/20 using eye exercises. Then a decade later he opened the Eye Gym in Los Angeles as a membership club for people who wanted coaching and practice in vision improvement strategies.

The Eye Gym was innovative and immediately popular, reports Gottlieb. A "visual work out" at the Eye Gym included trampoline jumping, eye relaxation techniques, Bates exercises, visualizations, chart work, self-massage, and psychological counseling, among other activities. "The Eye Gym was a brief but successful experiment," Gottlieb reflects today, noting that other professional demands forced him to close the facility a year or so after it opened.

In 1982 Gottlieb published an influential paper on the "Neuropsychology of Myopia," in which he surveyed existing theories on the cause of nearsightedness, then outlined his own "psychophysiological" model. His conclusion: nearsightedness results from habits of mental focusing and organizing mental processes to pay attention. This leads to chronic isometric contraction of the eye muscles, thereby elongating the eyeball. His prognosis: "Myopia is more flexible than is generally conceived."

Today he works with a psychotherapist in Manhattan on "Trampoline Intelligence Training." It's Gottlieb's practical way of instituting his principles of "psychophysical training." Gottlieb and other innovative optometrists including Kaplan use the trampoline in a variety of ways. They've developed exercises that can be performed on a gymnasium-style trampoline, with a smaller home-model, or even in your imagination. In the case of a real trampoline, a partner can call out reminders and instructions as you proceed.

The concept behind trampoline intelligence is that when you couple the rhythm of bouncing with visual tasks it rapidly hones attention, and this is the foundation for learning. Students jump in rhythm while being challenged to make quick, efficient visual decisions, like reading letters from a blackboard, interposing words, counting backwards, and moving the hands in the opposite direction to a series of arrows on a nearby wall chart. "You have to stay in a rapt attentive state to succeed at these visual tasks," comments Gottlieb.

The trampoline experience—dubbed "a leap toward learning"—is a microcosm of the learning process itself. It involves anxiety, emotional resistance, general body coordination, and strength of attention. When children do it, they learn how to pay attention in dynamic, flexible ways, rather than the habitual holding and contracting pattern most schoolchildren slide into.

According to Gottlieb, "This is the foundation of learning, involving coordination between visual and auditory systems, attention, and memory. The result is an integrated nervous system. Myopia comes from faulty habits of attention coupled with unresolved emotional tension. With psychophysical training like this as part of a child's basic educational process, we could develop high attention and healthy emotional responsivity and eliminate maybe 80 percent of future myopia."

Step Three: Overcome Emotional Obstacles

Become aware of how hidden emotions and basic psychological attitudes may hinder vision, and practice some of the mental exercises that can help you overcome psycho-emotional obstacles to better vision.

The process of visual recovery inevitably involves all aspects of the personality. Thus, by exploring your seeing habits you can gain a deep insight into your inner nature. According to vision therapist John Selby, "To understand how you see is to see yourself more clearly. Visual recovery is a whole body healing. You need a whole body program, with physical movement, emotional release, deep meditation, and spiritual opening." Learning how to see again, says Selby, involves not just some form of eye gymnastics, "but a deep spiritual restructuring of who you are in the world."

A number of other prominent vision therapists agree with Selby that personal and emotional factors can directly affect how you see. Jacob Liberman, O.D., for instance, is convinced that inner conflicts, compounded with breathing disorders and muscular-postural tensions, underpin vision problems. "Somebody gets myopic for a purpose, as a strategy, as a way of bringing the mind and body into some kind of different balance," he says.

Over the past thirty years psychologists and vision therapists have studied optometric patients and confirmed a link between personality traits and vision. The result is an intriguing composite model of the nearsighted and farsighted personality. According to Charles Kelley, Ph.D., founder of the Radix Institute of Ojai, Calif., and a leading figure in this field, the typical nearsighted person is withdrawn, emotionally controlled, and analytical. By comparison, the typical farsighted person is more often extroverted and gregarious.

Whether it's nearsightedness or farsightedness, "each eye condition is representative of a mind's eye perception," comments

Kaplan. "The present condition of the eye reflects past mind's eye pictures of how you saw parts of your world and life. It's a combination of your thoughts, beliefs, fears, and angers."

Vision therapists agree that the key is to identify emotions and fears that may be inhibiting your vision, and learn how to better ground yourself and express your true inner nature. A number of exercises, breathing techniques, and other practices can help you address these concerns in a way that can lead to better vision.

Fear of Seeing

"Many people do the Bates exercises until they're blue in the face but get no results," Selby says. "People who are successful with Bates have in conjunction moved into deeper spiritual spaces where healing takes place. It's more than just the physical eyes we need to heal to recover our vision. It's definitely possible to improve your vision naturally, but you need to see more clearly on all dimensions, not just the physical."

Thus, a person's general attitude and personality structure will be reflected in the way he or she performs certain visual functions, claims Selby. In particular Selby ties vision problems to early childhood fears. When prolonged, these fears become chronic anxiety. This fuels the emotional tendency to avoid the outside world, to reduce visual input to a minimum, and to shut yourself up in a myopic seclusion.

Selby posits different conditions leading to degrees of nearsightedness. High myopia—visual acuity of 20/200 or worse—he says is an emotional condition overlaid upon a genetic predisposition. He notes that in 80 percent of the cases he's seen, the severely nearsighted person experienced an emotional trauma around the age of 3-4, followed a few years later by an inhibition in self-assertion. The effect was to remove the vital flow of energy from the eyes, leading the child to hide his or her anger and mask emotional expression. Severe myopia then sets in around age 5-8.

On the other hand, Selby says, low myopia of 20/100 or better usually develops in early adolescence, between ages 10-14. Its typical cause is "a sexual-social fear of being seen."

Childhood thus is the ideal place to prevent myopia, says Selby.

When a child starts showing the symptoms of myopia, instead of automatically prescribing corrective glasses, why not inquire why the child no longer wants to see clearly. If we don't make this inquiry then, we're only deferring the crucial question until age 30 or 40.

By adulthood or midlife, the emotional difficulties are well structured into the body and have become a habit of seeing. At that time, one's entire posture blocks anger and withholds tension, says Selby, so that until the muscularly held psycho-emotional stress in the neck, shoulders, chest, and arms is resolved, the eyes will not release their blocked anger and distorted vision. Release can happen quickly. "If a person is willing to risk interacting through his eyes with the environment without glasses, I've seen the whole body posture shift in 30 seconds," Selby says.

Selby's convictions come partly from improving his vision from 20/100 to almost 20/20. He practiced Bates exercises for two years with no improvements before undertaking "bioenergetics" and "kundalini training," two mind/body practices that seek to release blockages of the vital energy that flows through the body. "This combination created an explosion inside me," he says. Within three weeks his acuity had dramatically and permanently improved. "I've spent the last 20 years," he says, "figuring out how it happened and how to reproduce this effect in others."

Liberman agrees that myopia isn't caused by heredity or even near-point stress in early schooling. Rather it's produced by cultural tyranny. "Kids are told to think but they're not allowed to express themselves emotionally," Liberman says. "They're told to control that energy. This produces contractions in the entire body. The eyes are only one portion of this body-wide contraction. Then when you add glasses to this, the whole balance has to compensate yet again. It's like putting a cast on your eyes for life. They never heal. Nor do the emotional issues ever get brought into the light of day."

For Liberman, there is not only a profound psycho-emotional aspect to wearing glasses, but a philosophical implication about how you put together your sense of the real world. "Glasses give you only a hard, sharp acuity, but you can't see peripherally very well with them; for that you need a soft focus. Usually the mind sees, separates, judges, and then instructs the eyes to look for the differences between things. We always see the figure against the ground. But when we practice viewing without glasses, with an open focus, not distinguishing the figure or the ground, but seeing both, shifting back and forth between them, we view without separation. Then we create unification in perception and this leads to unification in our inner being."

Liberman emphasizes full, unobstructed breathing as a major component of any vision improvement scheme. "The breath directly marries mind and body when it flows spontaneously. When we hold the breath this causes a separation of mind/body integration."

Meir Schneider, founder and director of the Center for Self-Healing in San Francisco, is living proof that radical improvement in vision is possible. As an adult, Schneider profoundly reversed the severe visual problems that had emerged during his infancy. He came to understand how as an infant he had concluded it was dangerous to see more things than ordinary children, and that persecution and punishment were the likely results. He says that this atmosphere of fear about seeing can permeate all the cells of your body, not just the eyes or brain. Thus, you must heal all the layers and change all the levels of patterning in the body, mind, and emotions, he counsels. Most nearsighted people can get rid of their glasses, he says, with the exception of those who developed myopia in their first two years of life. "It is physically possible but will take a lot of work," he adds.

Schneider says that when a young child experiences a strong negative emotion, such as fear, anxiety, frustration, rage, or humiliation, nearly always vision is temporarily worsened. If the experience is repeated and reinforced often enough, the visual impairment may become permanent. In the process, the child shifts from receiving the world with a soft eye to grabbing the world with a hard eye, explains Schneider. Emotional effects then become postural and these reinforce the visual impairment. "When you're frozen, trying to control the world, you become spastic in your eyes. Myopics tend to have a tight chest, for example, hold their backs tight, slope their heads forward. The tightness starts with looking forward, moving the neck and head forward to see, so the muscles freeze into this posture. The senses determine the posture, then this incorrect posture puts pressure on the eyes in a feedback loop."

Breaking Down the Eyes' Armor

This link between emotions, posture, and the eyes has been eagerly explored by bioenergetic practitioners such as Alexander Lowen, M.D., a pioneer of the body/mind field and the author of numerous books on emotions and health. For Lowen, the eyes are the expressive mirrors of the soul because they "directly and immediately reflect the energy processes of the body."

Lowen modeled his therapy, which includes exercises, bodywork, and other practices, on the work of the late Wilhelm Reich. A controversial psychoanalyst who tied bodily health to "orgone energy," Reich inspired a generation of bioenergetic healers such as Lowen to explore how psycho-emotional traumas can come to be mirrored in structures of the body.

According to bioenergetic analysis, the wide-eyed expression and mildly bulging eyeball characteristic of myopia is also the frozen look of fear. "The myopic eye is in a partial state of shock, thus blocking any emotion from registering in that organ," says Lowen. In his view myopia is a functional disorder or bodily distortion resulting from chronic muscular tensions. It needn't be irreversible. He says, "Many patients report some sustained vision improvement as a result of bioenergetic therapy."

The energetic basis for myopia is quite commonly first laid down in infancy or early childhood, usually involving an emotionally charged incident. Let's say a baby boy, in reaching out expressively with its eyes for a mother's love, sees anger or irritation instead. Lowen says that although the mother may be unaware of the expressive potency of her own eyes, "such looks by the parent are the equivalent of a fist in the face." The impact on the baby is to make him recoil in shock and contract his body. He may suppress his true feeling, intuiting a conflict between self-expression and survival. As shock and fear get structured into the eyes, vision is impaired and eyestrain and postural deformity begin. The muscles around the base of the head and jaw become contracted into a ring of tension that cuts off the flow of feeling to the eyes and maintains a state of chronic apprehension, explains Lowen. "This ring of tension is found in all cases of myopia. Psychologically the child retreats into a smaller, more confined space, shuttering out the disturbing elements in its world."

Lowen's analysis of the bioenergetic origin of myopia holds the key to its resolution. "Most important is to evoke the underlying fear so that it can be experienced and released." Among the basic exercises he uses for this purpose are diaphragmatic breathing, grounding, and the arch.

DIAPHRAGMATIC BREATHING. Lowen's first strategy is to raise a client's energy level through fuller and deeper breathing. As we'll see shortly in the discussion of myopic personality traits, commonly the breath is shallow, held, or constricted, and the diaphragm is tight. Lowen says, "Breathing has a positive effect on the eyes. After sustained deep breathing through the various exercises the eyes of most patients are noticeably brighter." Bioenergetic breathing is not about making yourself breathe but *letting* yourself breathe, Lowen emphasizes. His repertoire of bioenergetic exercises includes several for breathing.

BELLY BREATHING. Lie on your back on the floor, feet flat on the ground, knees up, legs 15 inches apart, the head back and neck extended. With your hands on the lower belly just above the pubic bones, breathe easily with the mouth open, observing the natural rise and fall of the abdomen. Practice for one minute. As a variation in the exercise of letting go, make a loud sound such as ah on the exhale and then try to maintain it for as long as possible without forcing it.

ROCKING THE PELVIS. While lying in the same position but with your hands on the ground, on the inhalation rock the pelvis forward, which means gently pull it (or roll it) back along the coccyx in towards the head. On the exhalation, roll it back out, as if gently pushing it away. Practice this exercise for one minute. Finally, lie on your back, arms extended along your side, palms down. Raise your legs until the heels are pointing toward the ceiling. Keep the knees bent and the feet flat out and pushing upward, parallel with the ceiling. Allow the breath to rise and fall spontaneously while in this position.

GROUNDING YOURSELF. Grounding, says Lowen, means pushing your center of gravity downward, out of the head, neck, and shoulders, so that there is a "feeling contact" between feet and the ground. Many people are often on their legs all the time, but rarely energetically in them. Once you're in your legs it's important to keep your knees flexed at all times and to let the belly out. These are the two postural commandments of bioenergetics, says Lowen. The "sucked in belly" makes free abdominal breathing difficult and inhibits emotional expression, both of which exert a restraining influence on eyesight.

Lowen coaches his clients into grounding through stages. First, stand with your feet 8 inches apart in a position that is posturally normal. Observe where your feet are, their orientation, the distribution of your body weight, your balance, and your vertical alignment. Then flex the knees slightly, make the feet parallel, and with your feet remaining flat on the ground, pitch your weight forward so that the balls of your feet carry it all. Bend and straighten your knees six times, then maintain the flexed position for 30 seconds.

Next, stand with your feet 10 inches apart, the toes turned slightly inward. While bending the knees a little, bend over forward to touch the floor with your fingers, letting your head hang loosely. Keep all your body weight on your feet, not the hands. Breathe without straining through the mouth. Hold for perhaps 30 seconds, then slowly rise up keeping the knees flexed. It's likely the leg muscles will vibrate and tingle. "This experience gives some idea of what grounding is about and that it is possible to sense one's self more fully in contact with one's base of support," says Lowen.

TAOIST ARCH. This exercise from the Chinese discipline of t'ai chi chuan is also recommended as "the fundamental stress position" by Lowen. He says, "A common problem I encounter in people is an overall body rigidity that doesn't let the person arch his body." Letting the belly out is a preliminary warm-up exercise to precede the arch. Stand with your legs about 8 inches apart, knees slightly bent, feet straight ahead and flat on the floor. Lean forward, putting all your body weight on the balls of your feet, while maintaining an erect but not stiff posture from the knees up. Let the lower abdomen out as far as it will hang while breathing easily through the mouth for a minute.

For the arch, stand with your feet 18 inches apart, toes turned slightly inward. Make your hands into fists and place them at the small of your back with the knuckles pointing upward. While flexing the knees and keeping the feet flat on the floor, arch your torso backwards over your fists while breathing deeply into your abdomen. Follow this exercise by doing another of the grounding exercises. This relieves postural stress, increases muscular flexibility, and helps discharge the "excitation" or energetic charge built up through the preceding exercises.

Self-reclamation and bioenergetic grounding can be a daunting experience at times, reminds John Barbaro, Ed.D., a bioenergetics practitioner at High Street Therapy Associates of Amherst, Mass., and one of about 1,200 bioenergetic analysts in the U.S. He recommends undertaking the therapy and exercises with the cooperation of a mentor or trained therapist for dialogue and counsel. There's a good psychological reason for this. "The issues interfering with one's ability to be free in one's life come through relating to other people," says Barbaro. If an individual initially registered the vision-inhibiting shock or fear from an emotionally-skewed moment of relation with a parent, then logically he or she needs to cathartically discharge this fright in relationship with another person, ideally a partner or therapist.

Lowen often directly helps a client release the blocked fear from the eyes by substituting himself for the offending parent while applying finger pressure to specific points on the face; frequently the result is a scream. Had the client screamed, for instance, at the time of being frightened by an angry glare and thereby dissipated the charge, there would have been no subsequent compensation for the shock through armoring of muscles, constricting of breathing, and shutting down of seeing. "You'll uncover fascinating things in your life, feel better about living, have more competency, and change your relationship with your eyes," says Barbaro. "Vision problems are an aspect of one's whole personality."

The Personality of the Eye

When strong emotions, posture, and vision remain locked in this feedback loop over time, definite personality traits become discernible, according to Kelley, another student of Reich. Kelley started with Bates exercises in 1946 to improve his nearsightedness, then 20/200 and 20/400. As he worked on his vision, Kelley realized that the basic Bates exercises failed to address or access deeper psychological issues and needed to be enriched with bioenergetic work. Kelley supplemented these exercises with inner emotional work founded on the principles laid down by Reich. In 1976 Kelley was able to boast that he had "lived normally for thirty years without the eye crutches."

In Kelley's view, the Bates method provided only a limited explanation of the way emotional and mental tension were translated into vision deficits. The primary source of the chronic eye tension which produces vision impairment is blocked emotion, said Kelley. Unless we free blocked emotions and feelings from the eyes locked in by ocular tension, a vision improvement program isn't likely to succeed.

In 1971 Kelley formulated his correlations of refractive error and Reichian body energy concepts. Each primary visual problem had a psycho-emotional signature, an armoring against the expression of a feeling, said Kelley. Myopia is blocked fear, hyperopia is repressed anger.

The myopic personality typically is withdrawn, introverted, detached, stubborn, emotionally controlled, and subject to daydreaming. The myopic is often sedentary and disinclined to take action, preferring contemplative activities such as reading. They're meticulous and somewhat fixated about time. For the myope, emotions require analysis and control, not action and expression.

Myopes prefer close-in, near-point activities where they feel visually comfortable in a small, tight space, often ignoring events or people in the distance. The myope prefers an occupation that emphasizes individual achievement such as scholar, architect, or journalist.

Physically, these traits tend to lead to a stiff neck and a chronically tense jaw that's rotated forward. The forehead is often cocked back and the shoulders forward and rigid. The chest may be depressed and the breathing shallow or blocked. The armoring of the eyes and the visual system is manifested as "a contraction and immobilization of all or most of the muscles of the eyeball, lids, forehead, and tear glands," says Kelley. The myopic often walks slightly hunched over, shoulders bent, the rib cage compressed, the abdomen tightened, and gaze on the ground. In essence, these are signs of armoring over a more fundamental inner fearfulness.

Myopia often emerges as an adaptive outcome from a feeling of vulnerability, as a psychological and perceptual protective barrier through which "out of sight" guarantees "out of mind." The myope fears seeing the future, the distant horizon, whether it's time or space, and pulls inward into himself. It's as if the myope repeats continually the negative affirmation: "I am afraid to see what's around me." The withdrawal of peripheral awareness becomes a form of perceptual defense.

The trouble is, all the choices comprising an individual's visual style become a self-supporting feedback loop. Myopia can produce lens bulge and make you seek out intense reading and near-point work, explains Edward Friedman, O.D., in *Dr. Friedman's Vision Training Program.* Myopes grow disinclined to follow non-reading activities and begin avoiding anything involving distance vision. "Slowly we can cut ourselves off from our general surroundings. This can lead to increased eye strain and progressively more severe nearsightedness," notes Friedman. The key point of course is that the myopic personality traits are usually so deeply embedded by the time you strap corrective lenses to your eyes that your artificially restored visual acuity doesn't dislodge these perceptual habits.

The behavior patterns and attitudes of the hyperope or farsighted person are also marked by a basic repression in energy expression, usually anger and rage. The behavioral profile of the hyperope is less thoroughly drawn, partly because optometrists regard myopia as an aberration, while a small amount of hyperopia is virtually normal. Hyperopes tend to throw temper tantrums and exhibit a discomfiting wildness. They're concerned with tomorrow, the horizon, the overall structure, with scanning the periphery. Most often extroverted and gregarious, hyperopes prefer team activities and careers such as public relations and business. Physically hyperopes are often erect and boardlike.

"My observation of hyperopes," comments vision therapist Janet Goodrich, "is that they are as over-controlled as myopes, but they are meeting authority with authority, rather than with fear."

Developing a New Visual Belief System

Goodrich includes bioenergetic work as well as other approaches in her teachings. She too came to the field after healing her own vision. An incessant reader, she suffered from severe nearsightedness as a child and first started wearing glasses at age seven. When she was twelve she read an article in a magazine about vision and became infuriated by the author's blithe dismissal of a nearsighted person's chances of ever eliminating glasses. Twenty years later Goodrich began adapting the protocols of Bates, Corbett, and Reich. In 30 months she was free of glasses. In 1967 she started to teach her "natural vision improvement" system and today she has trained and certified teachers in a half dozen countries.

For Goodrich the experience of reclaiming vision should be fun and easy. Emphasizing lifestyle changes rather than obligatory drills, she counsels students and trains teachers to work with the thought patterns that block seeing. She tells them to ferret out underlying vision inhibiting attitudes such as, "If I see clearly, I will be overwhelmed by demands."

"A psychological attitude with emotional affect or coloring is at the foundation of both impaired vision and good vision," Goodrich maintains. She agrees with Reich that when you block out your perceptions at any level of energy flow, the result is chronic muscular tension to keep it in place. "He knew thought patterns accompanied this, that visual memories were blanked out. To heal this you have to go back and relive those memories on all levels—physical, mental, and emotional."

Another powerful way to restructure your visual belief system is through self-hypnosis, according to vision therapist Lisette Scholl, author of *HypnoVision* and *Visionetics*. Scholl works with clients to change unconscious negative attitudes, ideas, and mental programs through self-hypnosis. "If you can't change your belief system, you can't change its control of your habits and functions," she notes.

Scholl discovered the efficacy of self-hypnosis after trying a variety of vision improvement techniques including Bates. After only six months, she had improved her vision somewhat. But when she "released my own deep-seated feelings of fearfulness" using self-hypnosis techniques, her vision made an impressive leap of clarity.

"Not only did hypnosis supply this long-sought-after missing link for vision improvement, but it is also the most powerful transformational tool I have ever encountered," Scholl says. Her teachings now combine Bates exercises and the restructuring of one's visual system through the unconscious.

Hypnosis works by deftly circumventing the objections of the conscious mind, explains Scholl. By skillfully planting affirmations and positive suggestions in the unconscious, you are powerfully and continuously reminding yourself to let go of the nearsighted or farsighted mindset. "The eye has an enormous capacity to physically change but it's hard to change these long-standing, deeply ingrained emotional and physiological habits unless we can get into that same unconscious level where your emotions are at work. Hypnosis gets us down to the core where we can assimilate a subject and make it our own. It's a gentle form of reprogramming. We put new habits in there as a precise form of positive affirmation. Then, as you free your vision, you'll free your whole being at the same time," Scholl says.

Exercises for Positive Eye Feelings

The following set of exercises and practices can help address these major visual issues of how to identify and release your fears and emotions, and assert your true self.

EYELOGUE JOURNAL. It's highly instructive to keep a daily record of your vision improvement program and the turbulent waters— thoughts, beliefs, fears, and angers—you might find leaping out of the depths of your retinas. From the mundane, such as which eye exercises you're doing, to the profound, such as psychological insights and realizations, the Eyelogue Journal provides "an invaluable source of feedback," according to Scholl, who first proposed it in *Visionetics*. Especially if you're an introspective myope, you may love this private dialogue with your eyes as you unravel a lifetime of attitudes, emotions, and thoughts about seeing. When I review the jottings in my Eyelogue about "canoeing the blur" and wearing my pinholes, I'm frequently inspired by the momentum and evident progress in understanding and practice that my daily entries reveal.

REBALANCING IDEAS. While the need for emotional healing is easily explained, the precise strategies less easily lend themselves to general formulation. Emotional release is usually a unique, even eccentric, self expressive experience, says Goodrich, who works regularly with clients individually and in groups to achieve this. As a preliminary exercise, group all your negative thought patterns about vision, seeing, competency, fear, inadequacy, blurriness, and progress, in your open left hand. List them, speak them out loud, and visualize them. Picture yourself, in terms of posture and expression, as you appear under their thrall. Then itemize the opposite, positive attitudes and affirmations, and similarly build them up in color, weight, size, and affect in your outstretched right palm. Now, as you overlap your hands in front of you, fuse both sets of attitudes, bring them together, merge and intertwine them, and wait for the psycho-emotional results. "People report it's no longer a big deal," says Goodrich. "The emotional content of resistance has melted away and they feel free."

The next phase of the psychological release exercise requires a partner or facilitator. This is what Goodrich does best at live workshops. She looks for the emotional thread, the shred of memory or inclination that, when pulled gently, can unravel a lifetime of visual suppression. She has the individual stand up, holding his body still while she stands next to him asking questions about his personal biography, his visual history, his inner attitudes, until something triggers his memory. She asks, for example, "What are your glasses protecting you from? How would you feel if somebody smashed them to pieces? Can you remember a time when you saw without them?" Goodrich reports that the student will often start to shake and perspire as he relives his childhood or some adult experience in which he had blocked, resisted, or judged what his eyes were perceiving. "They can't believe it but this happens every time," she says.

The next step is for Goodrich and the client to "celebrate" the resistance or judgment and find its opposite thought pattern. Goodrich helps the client identify positive attitudes: "If I see clearly I will grow expansive with vision. If I see clearly I will be able to express myself. If I see clearly I will be creative." Goodrich says, "Then we explore that possibility imaginatively, describing its contours and feelings. Sometimes that's more scary than the negative thought forms we're so used to." Finally, Goodrich inquires whether the client feels ready to choose to see better. "Choice makes a real difference in their lives," she says. "They are freed up within to do their vision exercises, to really *see* the trees and flowers and grass in the garden."

THE POSTURES OF FEAR AND ASSERTION. Selby suggests that the following exercise helps you to become aware of the difference in "excitation" or "charge" between a posture of fear and a posture of assertion. It also demonstrates how these postures affect your visual power and vitality.

First, assume the posture of fear, fright, and shock. Standing with your feet wide apart, inhale as you pretend something has frightened or surprised you. Watch as your knees lock up, your breathing tightens, your back arches, and your neck jerks your head upwards and backwards. Next discharge this fear vigorously. On the exhale, jump forward into a semi-squat, your knees bent, hands splayed across your knees, your head pitched forward, eyes and mouth wide open, and a growl of power issuing forth as you breathe fully out. Repeat the fear/inhalation phase, then jump forward again into assertion/exhalation.

AN EYEFULL OF GOOD INTENTIONS. It helps a great deal to affirm your positive intentions to see more, better, deeper, and wider. If unconscious attitudes and feelings hold your vision deficits in place as adaptive survival outcomes, why not change the tapes and rewrite the script? The idea is to modify your thinking consciously and deliberately through the constant repetition, in speaking and writing, of a positive intention and intended outcome. In a sly but radical way, this kind of willful talking-to-yourself can produce an inner shift in attitude and greatly aid your vision improvement program. In my case, an initial positive affirmation arose spontaneously while canoeing: "I give myself permission to see afar again." For the farsighted person Goodrich suggests the following: "My eyes are softly receiving the words and details of the close worlds, the inner worlds." For "transforming negatives" and "rebalancing your self-image" she recommends: "I am able to change. My eyes are ready for change. My eyes will respond. My eyes are able to see clearly at all distances." Kaplan suggests these: "My vision is improving every day. It is now okay for my eyes to see. My negative patterns of seeing are now dissolving. It is easy for me to recover my vision. My glasses are now becoming less a part of me."

PERSONAL POWER. This is a dynamic exercise in self-assertion that may access emotions underlying vision problems. It also enhances visual vitality, notes Selby.

First, stand with your feet wide apart. On a deep inhalation through the mouth, raise your arms over your head and tightly clench your fists while arching your back and bending your knees. Note any alteration in energy level or acuity in your eyes. On the exhalation through the mouth, bring your arms together and down as if to smash a table at waist-level. Be sure to flex your knees so that your torso remains upright. At the same time, make a sound on the exhale—*haaaiiiyaaahhh!*—as your tree-trunk-strong arms make contact with the imaginary table. Next time hold your breath for a moment before bringing down your arms and uttering the cry. Repeat six times, each time with more strength and speed—and with a smile, so you don't take the effect too seriously.

Step Four: Natural Remedies to the Rescue

Learn how to free the body's energy channels and treat minor vision problems using natural remedies that range from acupressure to herbs.

Natural healers seek to enhance the body's innate capacity for self-healing. Often the surest way to do this is to remove biochemical and physical obstacles to the natural flow of energy throughout the body. The life force or bodily energy goes by different names among the healing traditions, such as *qi* in Chinese medicine and *prana* in the medicine of India. Among the tools that these traditional healers use to balance and enhance the flow of life energy are techniques such as acupuncture, bodywork or self-massage, breathing exercises, and internal and external applications of healing herbs.

"When searching for the root cause of vision problems, we use the naturopathic trio of structure, chemistry, and energy," explains Ralph Wilson, a naturopathic doctor practicing at Spectrum Healing Arts in Lynnwood, Washington. Naturopaths are healers who use a variety of substances and techniques, including herbs, homeopathic remedies, and diet, to help the body regain its ability to get well. Wilson says that to resolve vision problems he routinely checks several areas of the body that Western medical scientists would regard as inconsequential to the function of the eyes. These areas include the liver, spine, and skull.

Traditional Chinese doctors also roam far from the eyes to improve vision. Oriental medicine and its practice of acupuncture describes twelve major bilateral energy pathways or "meridians" that traverse the body. Along with numerous other minor ones, these lines carry vital life energy or qi on behalf of primary organ systems. Five principal meridians have acupoints—points at or near the surface of the skin that can be needled or massaged to adjust the flow of energy—around the eyes.

More significant still for our understanding of the energy anatomy of the eyes, explains Raymond Himmel, an Oriental Medical Doctor and acupuncturist practicing in Mill Valley, Calif., is the fact that the major internal organs are closely allied with one of the five sense organs. The strongest ally of the eye is the liver. Himmel says, "The liver qi enters the back of the eye and spreads out through all the ocular tissues and muscles, the retina and iris."

Traditional Chinese healers typically use acupuncture, massage on acupoints ("acupressure"), or combinations of herbs to treat liver, eyes, and vision. In India the traditional medical techniques include massage, herbs, and yoga, the art and science of body positions and stretches for better health. Indian healers also pay particular attention to the quality of patients' breathing, which is closely linked with the well-being of the entire body as well as the ease and acuity of seeing. Special breathing exercises (*pranayama*) enhance the flow of prana and oxygen through the body.

Let's take a look at how traditional knowledge of the body's energy channels and some of these natural healing practices can help you to improve your vision.

The Body's Vision Points

Acupuncturists always look not only for the physical symptoms of a disease, but the underlying imbalance that causes the condition. Himmel says that deficits in vision and eye problems in this model are the symptoms, but the root cause is a diminishment of liver and possibly kidney energy.

Traditional Chinese medicine points to the liver because of the intimate energetic connections between that organ and eyesight, emotions, and the muscular system. The liver governs the free flow of energy throughout the body and generates all movement. This includes the circulation of qi, the discharge of digestive bile, and anything the moves you emotionally. The liver also governs the muscles and tendons and thus all anatomical movement.

Emotional states—tension, frustration, aggravation, irritability, anger, hysteria—negatively affect the liver, which then translates this aggravation into muscle and tendon spasms or contractions.

Most Americans' livers are additionally stressed from environmental and dietary toxins, including pollutants, alcohol, and drugs. The liver is the body's principal organ of detoxification, continually filtering the body's entire volume of circulating blood. And what doesn't stress the liver may negatively affect the kidney, the body's other systemic purifier. "Either way, stress on the liver and kidneys caused by these chemicals may contribute to a dysfunction in the eyes," says Himmel.

Early myopia in children aged 4-8 is most successfully treated with acupuncture and Chinese herbs, states Himmel. "With adults, if somebody has been myopic and worn glasses for years, the situation doesn't respond well to acupuncture. I've used acupuncture with better results on farsighted individuals just on the verge of needing reading glasses, or myopes who didn't want to 'progress' to bifocals."

CHINESE ACUPRESSURE MASSAGE. The acupuncture treatment of nearsightedness, farsightedness, and astigmatism is usually indirect, working energetically through the root meridians and not necessarily even near the eyes. Acupressure massage, however, involves gently pressing on various acupoints around the eyes. It can relieve eye tension, energetically stimulate the eyes, and fill them with healing qi. In many parts of China children practice acupressure eye massage regularly as part of their school curriculum to maintain eye health and prevent myopia. You can do it as a form of self-massage, or work with a partner.

Bates intuited the healing flow of energy through the body when he devised palming, comments Himmel. "We all have the ability to self-heal through our hands. There is a powerful energy point at the center of each palm. It's the place from which the Chinese qi gong masters send out energy. Putting that energy point over your eyes and doing a Bates visualization of blackness is a form of energetic palm healing that can have a powerful effect if you practice it every day."

Acupuncture treatment, acupressure massage, and Bates-type exercises make the best healing combination, suggests Himmel. "Acupuncture addresses the energy imbalances and speeds the process by bringing in more life energy to the eyes while the Bates

The following traditional Chinese acupressure massages are especially helpful for VDT operators and others who do extensive near-point work. They help to relax the eyes, increase blood circulation, and infuse the eyes with qi energy. Use a count of eight for each of the exercises, gently rubbing four times counterclockwise and then four times clockwise.

Resting four fingers lightly on the forehead, gently rub the point directly under the eyebrow with the thumb.

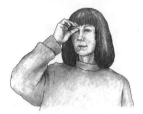 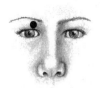

Use the thumb and forefinger of either hand to press and squeeze the points between the eyes near the base of the nose.

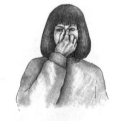 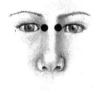

Supporting the chin with the thumbs, press and rub the points below the eyes using the forefinger and middle finger of each hand.

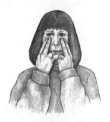 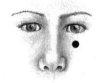

With fists against eyebrows and thumbs on temple, use the middle joint of the forefinger of each hand to rub points around the perimeter of the eyesocket.

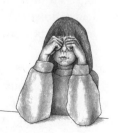 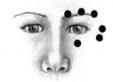

exercises help relax eye tension and reorganize the energetics of the ocular muscles."

Bodywork for the Eyes

A number of other points on the body, including the neck, shoulder, hands, and feet can also be massaged to benefit the eyes. For a shoulder and neck massage, the intent is not so much to directly stimulate acupoints but to palpate and relax the major muscles of this part of the body. Some degree of energy overlap would be expected, though.

A practice that has become increasingly popular in the U.S. is reflexology, which uses bodywork on the feet and hands to indirectly affect other parts of the body, including the eyes. Reflexologists contend that the hands and feet embody a complete map of the human body in miniature. Thus, massaging the appropriate point can stimulate an organ or a physiological process elsewhere in the body. For instance, massaging the right points on the feet can restore weak eyesight by helping to energetically balance the nerves and muscles of the eyes. Considering that the feet contain some 7,200 nerve endings that interconnect through the spine and brain with all regions of the body, this kind of energetic wiring isn't surprising.

SHOULDER AND NECK SELF-MASSAGE. Sit comfortably in a chair with your feet on the floor. Raise your arms above your head, stretch and inhale deeply, then lower them, bending at the elbows and placing your hands on your back as far down as they'll go. The fingers of each hand face in towards the spine. Press firmly into the muscles with your fingertips, gradually moving up the sides of the spine (don't press on the vertebrae but alongside them) to the base of the neck. Let your head gradually fall forward. Repeat three times. Next take your right hand and locate a point on the left shoulder muscle near the base of your neck. This pea-sized point will be tender, possibly stiff and sensitive. Press and vibrate your right index and middle finger into this point for 10 seconds, then use your left hand to massage the right shoulder point.

With both hands back on the base of the neck, move the thumbs in a circular motion to massage the hollows on either side of the spinal column at the base of the skull. Next slowly move your fingers up the skull and the thumbs across the base of your skull towards the ears. Your thumbs may encounter three sensitive spots along the way which can take extra but gentle thumb stimulation. Massage your scalp with all five fingers and let your jaw fall open in relaxation. Massage your entire face with your fingertips, applying gentle but firm pressure and circular motion across its entire surface. For example, trace the musculature of the jaw from ear to throat, then the space between ear and eye socket, then eye socket and mouth. After 10 minutes of this meticulous self-massage your face quite likely will feel warm and tingling.

FOOT REFLEXOLOGY MASSAGE. The eye points are located in a thin strip at the base of the second and third toe on the bottom of each foot. Reflexologists point out that quite commonly a person with weak eyesight will register tenderness or soreness in these points. Reflexology foot massage is a simple practice you can perform on your own feet or can enjoy receiving from a partner.

For self-massage, sit on a chair or the floor and cross your legs so that you can reach the feet. Find the base of the second and third toes where they meet the puffy ridge of the metatarsal padding. Press with both thumbs, moving laterally along this ridge. For massaging a partner, place your thumb at the base of the metatarsal ridge and your other four fingers on the front side of the foot. Move your thumb up and down the eye point strip, pressing in firmly. Other points to stimulate that may help the eyes include the neck nerve reflex point (work your thumb down the outside and inside edges of the big toe to its base) and the kidney and liver reflex points in the midpoint of each sole.

The hand also contains a complete reflexology map of the body. In fact, according to Korean acupuncturist Tae Woo Yoo, it contains a complete miniature acupoint meridian system as well. Also, the hands are easier to self-massage than the feet.

HAND REFLEXOLOGY MASSAGE. The eye points are located at the base of the four fingers of both hands on both sides. To self-massage the left hand, place your right index finger on an eye point on the palm side of your left hand and your thumb on the opposite (back) side. Rub each point vigorously for a minute or so and then reverse for the right hand.

"By working the eye reflexes I won't promise that you are going to be able to throw your eyeglasses away," comments reflexologist Dwight C. Byers, author of *Better Health With Foot Reflexology.* "What I am saying is that if the eyes are growing weaker, you may be able to prevent further deterioration and not have to change your eyeglasses as often."

Breathing for Eye Health

Another route to improving the flow of energy to and from the eyes is through the breath. In Step Three we saw how bioenergetic healers work with the breath to access emotional states that can affect vision. Breathwork such as through yoga can also help detoxify the body by expelling carbon dioxide. The overall effect is to strengthen the nervous system, improve blood circulation, calm the mind, and stimulate the eyes.

As a therapy, yoga works best when it's adjusted to the medical and health needs of the individual, explains Richard Miller, Ph.D., a yoga instructor for over 20 years and a co-founder of the International Association of Yoga Therapists. The goal, Miller says, is "the precise application to the individual of different yoga modalities, including postures, breathing, prayer, and meditation. You can't give a generic prescription without seeing the individual because there can be ten different causes for the complaints of ten different people. Each person needs a different prescription." Notwithstanding, Miller says that the following pranayama exercises can complement most vision improvement programs.

The sitting posture for all of the following exercises is the same. Sit in a chair with your feet on the floor, or kneel on the floor with your knees six inches apart and your buttocks resting on a pillow propped on your heels. Even better if you can do it is to sit cross-legged on the floor with your back straight, knees touching the floor, and hands in your lap.

COOL BREATHING. This breathing exercise soothes the eyes and ears, activates the liver, and lowers blood pressure slightly. Assume position. Open your mouth, make an "O" with your lips, and stick your tongue out over your teeth and past your lips. Inhale through the mouth, sucking in air over the tongue as if through a narrow straw. After a full inhalation, close your mouth and hold the breath for five seconds. Place your right index finger or thumb on the side of your right nostril to block it and exhale slowly through the left nostril, prolonging it as much as possible without straining. Repeat, alternating nostrils on the exhale, for five minutes.

SUBTLE ENERGY BREATHING. This breathing exercise cleanses the subtle energy channels throughout both hemispheres of the brain, purifies the nerves, and calms the mind. Assume position. Close both eyes and concentrate on your left eye. Observe its sensations and try to bring it alive with feeling. Inhaling through the nostrils, flood your left eye with prana. Even better, imagine your left eye is a nostril capable of drawing in air. As you exhale, transfer alive feeling from your left eye to your right one. Then reverse, inhaling aliveness through the right eye, transferring it to your left eye, and exhaling while concentrating on the left eye. Repeat this sequence for five minutes.

Next, take your left index finger and block the left nostril by pushing on its side. Inhale slowly and steadily but not forcibly through the right nostril to a count of three, five, seven, or more if comfortable. Imagine your right eye is simultaneously inhaling and receiving oxygen and prana. Then unblock your left nostril, block your right one, and exhale slowly through the open left nostril to a count of six, ten, fourteen, or more (double the count of the inhalations). Imagine this time your left eye is the recipient of alive sensations. Then inhale slowly through the left nostril, block it, unblock the right nostril, and exhale slowly through it. Practice this sequence for five minutes.

LUSTROUS SKULL. This exercise features rhythmic contractions of the diaphragm and vigorous exhalations. It activates and invigorates the liver, pancreas, spleen, and abdominal muscles, improves digestion, drains the sinuses, makes the eyes feel cool, and generally produces exhilaration. This exercise, however, is not recommended for anyone with a detached retina or glaucoma.

Assume position. Inhale deeply but not forcefully though the nose. On the exhale contract your diaphragm by pulling it up and in, forcefully expelling air through the nostrils like a bellows being closed shut. Let the abdomen relax outward for a second, then repeat. Set up a steady rhythm of these "bellow" exhalations. Try this exercise for 20 rounds, rest for a few minutes, then do another round of 20. If you feel dizzy before you finish any of the 20 rounds, stop, relax, and breathe calmly before resuming.

BREATHING WITH THE GRAIN. This is breathing in regular gradations and orderly succession, by inhaling through both nostrils but exhaling alternately through either nostril. A nerve and sense purifier, it also relaxes and softens the diaphragm, stimulates the parasympathetic nervous system but calms the sympathetic, and slightly lowers blood pressure.

Assume position. Inhale deeply through both nostrils. Hold your breath for 5-10 seconds. Block the left nostril with your left index finger and partially block your right nostril with your right index finger. Exhale long and slowly through the right nostril. Next, inhale long and deeply through both nostrils, holding your breath as before. But this time block the right nostril and partially block the left nostril. Exhale long and slowly through the left nostril. Practice 5-8 cycles.

The Vision Herbs

Both Western and Oriental herbal traditions specify a handful of herbs or herbal combinations that can positively affect vision. Generally, the Western herbs are taken in the form of a capsule or tea, or administered as a compress. They are most effective in promoting night vision, for instance, or treating specific eye complaints, such as sore, inflamed eyes. The Chinese apothecary, on the other hand, is more exotic in its concoctions and ambitious in its claims. There is even, for instance, a "myopia pill" patent medicine available.

Most reputable herbalists refrain, however, from claiming that either Western vision herbs such as bilberry and eyebright, or Oriental patent medicines, will directly improve nearsightedness or farsightedness. These conditions are usually too entrenched for the specific action of herbs. What herbs can do is energetically support the health of the eyes, either through detoxifying and strengthening organs such as the liver and kidneys or by enhancing the overall energy of the body. In either case, the herbs' action can support other vision improvement efforts you're making, such as exercising the eyes or eating an optimum diet.

While the therapeutic use of herbs is empirically well-established it would be prudent to first consult a Western herbalist or Oriental medicine expert on the exact matching of their apothecaries with your individual vision condition.

BILBERRY. Also known as blaeberry, whortleberry, and huckleberry, bilberry (*Vaccinium myrtillus*) came to prominence during World War II when British RAF pilots consumed bilberry jam before night missions. Subsequent scientific research has substantiated their claim and the advice of folk healers that bilberry temporarily improves night vision and visual acuity. The active ingredient is apparently certain flavonoids called anthocyanosides. These are found in concentrations of only 0.1-0.25 percent of the fresh bilberry fruit, and for healing purposes are much more concentrated in herbal preparations.

Scientists say that the anthocyanosides apparently have a salutary effect on enzymes essential for vision (including rhodopsin) and stimulate the retina's dark-adapted rods, essential to night vision. Western herbalists also recognize bilberry's effectiveness in providing temporary relief for chronic eye fatigue (such as from prolonged reading), day blindness (hemeralopia), and certain vascular disturbances of the retina. Bilberry's therapeutic influence (after a dose of 25-50 mg) peaks for four hours then wanes away for the next twenty.

Bilberry is available, either alone or in combination with other herbs, in capsule or tablet form (with 15-25 percent anthocyanosides) from several U.S. herbal distributors. Most natural foods stores with a varied herbal section carry it.

EYEBRIGHT. Another vision herb native to Europe with a long history in Western herbology is eyebright (*Euphrasia officinalis*). It's used in the form of an eye lotion for conjunctivitis, or as a capsule or tea to reduce eyestrain and clear and restore the eyes. Herbalists also use eyebright for acute or chronic eye inflammations, stinging or weeping eyes, and hypersensitivity to light. While scientists are uncertain how eyebright's active chemical constituents (such as glycosides, tannins, alkaloids, and essential oils) exert their effect—or if they have significant therapeutic merit at all—many herbalists embrace eyebright.

To make an infusion, pour one cup of boiling water into a china or glass teapot containing 1 teaspoonful of dried eyebright or 3 teaspoons of the fresh herb. Put a lid on and let steep for ten minutes before straining and drinking.

Eyebright is also effective when applied topically, as an eye compress. To make a compress, first make an infusion or a decoction. The latter is made by adding one teaspoonful of dried eyebright to one cup of water in a pot, bringing the mixture to a boil, simmering for ten minutes, straining, and then allowing the liquid to cool slightly. Immerse and soak a palm-sized piece of clean cloth, made of cotton, linen, or gauze, in the eyebright infusion or decoction. Wring out the cloth slightly, tilt your head back, and place the compress over half-open eyes (the compress shouldn't be in direct contact with the lens of the eye) for fifteen minutes or until the cloth cools.

Like bilberry eyebright is also available in capsule form in most natural foods stores. Many herbal companies combine eyebright with other herbs, such as goldenseal root, bayberry bark, and red raspberry leaves to make a tonic that contributes minerals, vitamins, and enzymes useful to the eyes.

Herbal tea bag compresses are an intriguing, instant option. Moisten teabags containing chamomile, fennel, parsley, or eyebright tea and place on each open eye for five minutes. Or make an herbal eyewash using 1 tablespoon crushed fennel seed, 1 tablespoon crushed comfrey root, and 10 ounces of water. Boil the mixture, cool, and strain off the herbs. Bathe the eyes using a glass eyecup.

ORIENTAL HERBS AND CHINESE PATENT MEDICINES. In many respects the pharmacopeia of Oriental medicine has far more specific and potent herbal remedies available for treating vision problems and generally enhancing visual capability. The following list includes various "vision improving formulas" usually in pill form available through Chinese specialty food stores, Oriental pharmacies, or mail-order herbal suppliers (see Resources). Often their pharmaceutical description is presented in the traditional jargon of Oriental medicine and acupuncture energetics.

Gardenia and Vitex Combination (in Chinese, *Xi Gan Ming Mu Tang*) contains 19 herbal ingredients that benefit the eyes by "dispelling wind and heat" that produce eye disorders.

Chrysanthemum Combination (*Zi Shen Ming Mu Tang*) is a 15-ingredient mixture including ginseng, licorice, and angelica that tonifies qi, cleanses the liver, and nourishes the kidneys, all of which benefit the eyes.

Lycium, Chrysanthemum, and Rehmannia Formula (*Qi Ju Di Huang Wan*) contains 27 percent rehmannia root and seven other herbs that nourish the kidneys, replenish the blood, and strengthen the liver. It works to heal eye disorders such as blurred vision, dryness, pain, and photosensitivity due to "liver and kidney yin deficiency."

Bright Eyes Upper Clearing Tablets (*Ming Mu Shang Qing Pian*), 12-component pills (50 percent of which is gardenia fruit and angelica), sedate liver fire that negatively affects the eyes by causing redness, itching, tearing, and conjunctivitis.

Inner Obstruction to Eyesight Pills (*Nei Zhang Ming Yan Wan*) contain 16 herbs that encourage visual clarity, "nourish liver and kidney yin," and relieve vision impairment due to "liver yin deficiency with heat" (with symptoms of cataract, glaucoma, or itchy, painful eyes).

Dendrobrium Leaf Night Sight Pills (*Shi Hu Ye Guang Wan*) contain 18 ingredients (including 16 percent ginseng) and are prescribed to nourish the qi and blood and tonify the liver and kidney. They can aid blurry or dizzy eyesight, hypertensive intraocular pressure, and dry eye, and are especially valuable in the early stages of cataracts.

Bright Eyes Rehmannia Pills (*Ming Mu Di Huang Wan*) contain 12 ingredients (18 percent rehmannia root and 7 percent chrysanthemum) that replenish liver and kidney, nourish blood, "sedate liver fire and wind," and thereby aid the eyes.

Other Natural Remedies for Vision

Naturopath Ralph Wilson routinely checks a new client for liver status, particularly if there is an accompanying vision problem or even "normal" nearsightedness, farsightedness, or presbyopia. Exposure to environmental, dietary, and household pollutants that overstress and toxify the liver must be eliminated before vision can be permanently improved, advises Wilson. Further, chronic constipation can create a negative feedback loop with the liver and eyes. Intestinal microbes putrefy undigested, unexcreted protein matter in the large intestines producing bowel toxemia. The toxins get absorbed in the blood and circulate through the liver for detoxification, but if the liver is already stressed, this additional burden may render it partially dysfunctional. The end result is that the eyes and eyesight suffer. Hence bowel purgatives, laxatives, enemas, and liver detoxifiers are often recommended.

The 200-year-old medical science of homeopathy seeks to treat "like with like." In other words, homeopaths use extremely minute doses of substances that in larger quantities would tend to induce the symptoms that the homeopath is trying to relieve. Wilson, who has training in homeopathy, says, "In the case of a vision problem, I would look for an appropriate homeopathic constitutional remedy to strengthen the body's underlying immune defense and repair system, remove stress on the body, and provoke and clarify fundamental underlying physical and psychological issues."

According to the protocols of classical homeopathy, a generic prescription for vision problems, whether defects in acuity or eye diseases, isn't possible and wouldn't be correct practice. Homeopathy is quintessentially individual case prescription based on an individual's unique psychophysical constitution. Nor does homeopathy prescribe a remedy to an individual for a single, specific symptom, such as conjunctivitis. It's a question of taking the entire case and treating the whole person. It wouldn't be unusual, however, for a vision problem to eventually improve over the course of several months of homeopathic treatment. Homeopathy is best at resolving deep-set conditions that underlie many organic complaints and difficulties. Obviously, nearsightedness and farsightedness will be part of that overall symptom picture.

A somewhat related natural therapy potentially useful for correcting vision problems makes use of the essences of flowers and herbs. The underlying concept is that within the plant world there are numerous curative correlations between botanical essences and human emotions or psychological states. The plant kingdom in a sense is a therapeutic repertory for human psycho-emotionality. Thus flower essences can creatively support positive, wholesome changes within you as you move toward greater well-being on all levels, according to Patricia Kaminski, co-director of the Flower Essence Society of Nevada City, Calif.

"We've had some success in vision improvement through treating for overall stress reduction," Kaminski says. "We treat the person, not the illness. We'll treat someone who has fear, tension, or stress, factors which are larger than the vision problem alone. We have noted that when we work with a vision problem at an early stage of onset, in childhood, it's a lot easier to use flower essences to access the emotions."

Kaminski tells how flower essences helped a troubled 8-year-old boy who was hyperactive, prone to yelling and acting out, dyslexic, uncooperative, and nearsighted. His favorite fantasy was that he was a spaceman reluctantly living on Earth. In working with him, the practitioner suggested the essences shooting star (a wild sister to cyclamen, used as a "rebirthing" essence for people who haven't "connected with physical life"), wild rose (to treat "disengagement and a lack of enthusiasm and caring"), and chamomile (a typical remedy for hyperactivity). After three months, the boy experienced remarkable improvements in schoolwork, reading ability, and attitude, and no longer needed glasses.

Flower essence therapy works best when it's individually tailored. But you can self-prescribe based on the published repertoire available from the FES, creators of more than six dozen subtle flower essence preparations. The FES also maintains an informal U.S. network of about 3,000 flower essence practitioners, including nurses, chiropractors, bodyworkers, and psychics. Additionally, there are other flower remedy systems available, including the original Bach Flower Remedy system, 38 essences developed by the English physician Dr. Edward Bach in the 1930s.

Step Five: Free the Body to See

Become conscious of how movement, posture, and alignment of head, neck, and torso can affect vision, and use exercises and adjustments to correct patterns that can impair better vision.

I recently had lunch with a man who spoke animatedly with his whole body. The thoughts and sentences rolled out of him while his body described a fluid ballet of emphatic gestures. He raised his arms, rolled his wrists, snapped his fingers, stood up, and pointed. His sparkling brown eyes roamed the room, the table, my face, flashing meaning and presence. I couldn't help but notice that my friend wasn't wearing corrective lenses. I questioned him about his vision, and he described his eyesight as sharp and healthy.

Later I wondered more about the possibility of a link between his vision and his free and expressive movement, the way he held and carried himself so wonderfully. Could the impact of corrective lenses on spatial relationships, depth perception, and other visual factors be felt and seen in the body? Is there a clear relationship between one's visual world and a person's style and sense of movement, expression, and even posture? Emphatically yes, say many practitioners not only of vision therapy but various body-work and movement disciplines, including Rolfing, Alexander Technique, and Feldenkrais work.

Vision-aware chiropractors, yoga teachers, and other practitioners agree that if you're beginning to take steps to improve your vision after longtime use of corrective lenses, you may be carrying your head too far forward on the spine, or your neck may be tilted or cocked to the side. You may also be moving your neck, head, and torso in improper ways, be constricted in your breathing, or be tense. By addressing these concerns, you can free the eyes to attain their natural power.

Aligning Head, Neck, and Torso

From my own experience I now suspect that my chronic neck problems are related if not reinforced by my nearsightedness. When I put my glasses back on after an hour of not wearing them, almost involuntarily my neck stiffens up and muscular tension encircles my head. Which comes first, the myopia or the neck problem, is difficult to say, but that they work together in "a vicious cycle, a continuous feedback loop," is certain, according to Jan M. Jensen, D.C., of the Jensen Chiropractic Center in Milwaukee.

"If the cervical vertebrae of the neck are out of alignment, this affects the balance of the head on the neck and the orientation of the eyes," explains Jensen. "If the upper neck is out of alignment, the cranial bones become microscopically misaligned, too. The myopic person characteristically tilts the head forward, making it easy for the neck to go into subluxation."

Subluxation is a key term for chiropractors. It means something less than (or sub-) a full-blown joint dislocation, and refers to any malpositioning, abnormality of movement, or compression between neighboring vertebrae in the spinal column. With a subluxation, nerves get pinched or stretched by the displaced vertebral bones, the inter-vertebral discs get compressed, and the flow of what chiropractors call "the vital nerve force" is disrupted. This impairs the free circulation of oxygen, nerve stimulus, and energy into the brain and eyes.

Chronic, untreated subluxations disrupt the body not only by hampering movement but by impairing normal physiological functions such as respiration or digestion. "The worst kind of subluxation is of the sphenoid bone in the skull," explains Jensen, "because this puts pressure on the eyes and directly causes astigmatism."

It's sometimes possibie to tell if a cervical, thoracic, or lumbar vertebra is subluxated because there is usually some physical discomfort, such as a tender spot on the spine or a painful tightness in a muscle. A fixation, which is a cluster of misaligned, fused vertebrae, is harder to self-detect but may be more injurious to long-term spinal integrity. Fixations commonly produce numerous "referred pain" patterns elsewhere in the body.

There are simple body signs to look for that may alert you to potential subluxations or fixations, advises Jensen. The signs are easier to find if a friend or partner helps out.

• Probe your spine for tender, hot spots.

• Notice if your shoulders are uneven when standing erect.

• Check for tightness in the upper neck where it meets the skull, or restrictions in lateral movement.

• Examine your head to see if it tilts or seems crooked with respect to the vertical orientation of your neck.

• Examine the bottom tips of your earlobes against a sheet of gridpoint paper to see if they're level.

If your vertebral alignment isn't what it could be, some of the following exercises or a series of chiropractic adjustments may help you reclaim your vision.

"It makes any vision therapy program go that much easier," claims Jensen, who improved her own vision using chiropractic and Bates-style exercises. "The combination often produces great results. I've seen it clear up headaches, eyestrain, and glaucoma."

According to Michael Copland-Griffiths, D.C., president of the British Chiropractic Association and author of *Dynamic Chiropractic Today*, the following exercises "can be performed by almost all chiropractic patients with the minimum of risk." If any exercise produces dizziness, light-headedness, or pain, discontinue, says Copland-Griffiths. He also suggests that the neck exercises not be performed without the approval of a chiropractor because they might aggravate a cervical subluxation.

RAINBOW NECK. While sitting comfortably and erect in a chair, cross your arms to temporarily lock the thoracic spine. With your eyes open, imagine a stunning rainbow spans the horizon before you. Turn your head to see the lower left base of the rainbow where it dissolves into the ground. Then trace its chromatic striations up to the peak of the arch. Let your eyesight flow with the curving colors down the righthand arc to the ground. Allow your head to relax and droop. Reverse this procedure from right to left, and repeat a few times. "The aim is to carry your neck through a composite of movements that will exercise it without over-reaching," explains Copland-Griffiths.

NECK MOBILIZATION. This is a three-step neck exercise that you can practice sitting or standing. First, bend your head forward slowly so that your chin approaches your chest. Bring your head only as far forward and down as feels comfortable—don't strain or force it. Then reverse, slowly and gently drawing the head backwards toward your spine. Again, do not strain. Repeat. Next, keeping your head facing forward tilt it to the right as far as it will comfortably extend, trying to press your ear to your shoulder. Reverse the movement toward the left shoulder, and repeat. Last, without raising your shoulders, slowly and gently rotate your head to the right as if to look over your shoulder at something behind you. Hold this position for 5 seconds, then reverse, rotating your head to look behind your left shoulder. Hold for 5 seconds, then return to your original position. Try repeating this sequence a few times.

CHICKEN WALK. This exercise, which mimics the way a chicken bobs its beak and head, stretches the joint between the base of the skull and the top of the spine. While sitting or standing, look straight ahead at an object perhaps 4-6 feet from your face. Fix your eyes on this object, then push your head forward keeping your chin up. Extend the head forward only as far as feels comfortable. Then retract it, pushing back as far as possible within your range of comfort.

ISOMETRIC NECK STRENGTHENERS. This series of exercises strengthens the neck muscles by tensing them against a resistance. Breathing calmly, place your hands on your forehead and then push your head downward against their resistance. Hold for a count of 5, relax, then repeat. Interlock your fingers behind your head at the back of your skull. Push gently against this hand hold, count to 5, release, and repeat. Next, raise your arms and place your palms against your ears as if to block out sound. Press your head to the right as if to press your ear to the shoulder but use your right hand to prevent any movement. Hold this resistance for five seconds, release, and then repeat in the opposite direction. Finally, move your palms slightly off the ears toward your eyes, splay the fingers out over the forehead, and hook the thumbs under the earlobes. Try to move your head to look over your right shoulder while your hands restrain your head from moving. Hold this for 5 seconds, release, then reverse the isometrics to the left.

The next exercise is not from the chiropractic tradition but rather a useful adaptation from hatha yoga that can not only improve eyesight but "align your head with your spine and release the flow" of toxins, comments Earlyne Chaney in *The Eyes Have It*. This exercise is not recommended for anyone with neck problems.

FORWARD NECK STRETCH. Sit on a bench or broad chair with your feet on the ground about 18 inches apart and your posture erect but relaxed. Bending at the waist, drop your head between your legs, allowing your neck to stretch. Lift your chin to look toward the ceiling, but only as far as feels comfortable. Release your neck and allow your head to dangle between your legs again. Sitting upright again, try to touch your left ear to your left shoulder, then your right ear to your right shoulder. Move your neck only as far as feels comfortable. Return your head to its relaxed dangling position. Sitting up, rotate your head to look over first your right and then your left shoulder. Return to the resting position.

Sitting up again, interlock your fingers behind your neck at the nape. Inhale, then bend slowly forward and lower your head to between your legs. Exhale vigorously. Allow your fingers gently to press your head a little further downward, encouraging your neck to stretch. Again, do not strain or over-stretch. Hold for a few seconds, then release and return to an upright position.

Getting Your Body Organized

Postural and structural support for vision recovery is also available through Rolfing, the deep massage therapy founded by biochemist and physiologist Ida Rolf (1896-1979). Rolf said that although her system was not specifically designed to improve eyesight, "Vision is usually changed for the better following Structural Integration [Rolfing]."

Rolf viewed glasses as artificial aids to vision that immobilize the eyes and prevent exercise of the muscles that control focusing. "This lack of physical exercise gives the starved, toneless appearance characteristic of eyes that always look through glasses," she said. "In the eye, as in all other parts of the body, movement translates into vital life; immobility shifts us toward the apathy that eventually becomes death."

Rolfing's aim is to better organize the body's structure. Rolfers do this by manipulating the fascia, an intricate web of connective tissue around muscles and bones. Fascial tone and elasticity, explains Jeffrey Maitland, a practitioner and faculty chairman at the Rolf Institute of Structural Integration in Boulder, Colorado, are basic contributing factors in our overall well-being. If one segment of this fascial web is "thickened" or disorganized, it transmits strain throughout the body the way a snag in a sweater distorts the overall weave.

"A lot of vision problems are rooted in deep tension in the neck, cranium, eyes, and upper back," says Maitland. "But unlike chiropractic, we manipulate the strain patterns of the soft tissues. Then the spine starts to line up properly and the bones go where they belong."

Observe a person walking down the street, says Maitland. You'll note that many people carry their heads too far in front of their body, somewhat like elderly people walking hunched over. This habit struggles against an instinctive reflex to right our posture and cranial position to get our eyes looking straight out. "So no matter how twisted your body is or how much your head leans far forward, you'll do everything to put your eyes straight," says Maitland. This is postural survival at all costs, but it's not the formula for healthy vision.

If you go to one of the 600 trained Rolfers in the U.S., expect to have at least 10 sessions devoted to achieving the principal goal of "getting your body organized," Maitland says. "If you came in with chronic neck problems and poor vision, before I could get your neck or head straight, I'd have to get your legs and feet properly under you. Otherwise any adjustments you get in your neck or spine wouldn't last.

"I've seen Rolfing improve vision, as all Rolfers have, but it doesn't happen with such regularity that we can say, 'vision improvement is part of what Rolfers do.' Many people tell us that after a Rolfing session their vision seemed more acute or colors more brilliant."

Acuity isn't the totality of vision nor is its recovery the final touchstone of success, Maitland, who wears glasses, reminds us. He used Rolfing and meditation to deepen his perception. "I went from just looking at things to being able to truly see. Perception is much bigger than looking with our eyes. Perception is a whole body phenomenon."

Improving Body Use and Movement

If perception is a whole body phenomenon, you need to become more aware of how you use your body in various activities. Through conscious effort, it is possible to identify how imbalances in the relationship of the head and neck to the torso generate breathing difficulties, spinal distortion, and tension. You can then eliminate action and movement habits that are inefficient or cause tension. That's the line of thinking in the Alexander Technique, a practitioner-assisted approach to better posture and movement formulated almost a century ago by the Australian actor Frederick Matthias Alexander (1869-1955).

Alexander practitioners train clients in the subtleties of self-observation and movement awareness. "My job is to get you to see what you're actually doing with the way you use your body," explains Michael Fredericks of Ojai, Calif., one of about 300 trained Alexander instructors in the U.S. "Use" for Alexander practitioners refers to the quality and habits of movement, patterns of reacting to stress, and ways of holding the head and neck with respect to the torso. By correcting use, we regain "primary control."

The Alexander Technique, like Rolfing, doesn't go straight for the eyes. You can't change habits of incorrect use starting with the individual part, notes Fredericks. "Tension in a part, like the eyes, can be a reminder to you to come back to an observation of your total way of using yourself," he says. He believes that eye exercises and other vision improvement strategies are useful, but if at the same time "you're creating excess stress in the way the whole body works, it's like trying to bale water out of a sinking boat using a colander."

According to Fredericks, "It's a matter of looking at your physical habits and developing a discipline of postural self-awareness. It takes a while to learn because you're dealing with strong habit patterns while learning a new language." For example, he says, how do you see? Is it with a kind of tunnel vision, pushing toward what you see, or are you receptive in the sense of allowing what you're looking at to come to you?

"We demonstrate in your body what freedom in the relationship of head, spine, and torso is like," says Fredericks. "You experience, for instance, how the head can be freely poised on the top of the spine, without narrowing the shoulders into a slump. You begin releasing that pattern of interference connected to the tension in seeing. You no longer lock in with your vision, creating interference patterns with your head, neck, spine, and torso."

"The technique is concerned with how you do anything in a coordinated way, even how you do Bates eye exercises," explains Alex Murray, an instructor with the North American Society of Teachers of the Alexander Technique in Champaign, Illinois. Murray points out, "If the vision exercises you do are at the expense of your total pattern of good use, you're setting yourself up for problems in the future."

The Alexander re-education of body use doesn't happen overnight. The standard recommendation is 30 lessons, starting with two per week for the first two months. Like Rolfing, it's practitioner-dependent, although it does assign the client some home practice. Once you gain awareness of what good use and natural coordination feel like, Fredericks says that the basic instruction is to ask yourself, while doing anything, "How can I be easier within this activity? What am I doing in this activity that's creating excess tension or stress?"

According to Fredericks, not only can we constructively observe our own patterns of use, we can objectively note the habits of movement of others. Watch how they move, how they interfere in their moving by slumping, how they create stress as they move through space, advises Fredericks. "When you see this without judging, use this as a wake-up call to look at yourself. Are you creating tension by jacking your shoulders up around your ears when you carry that box? Can you let go of that tension pattern and come back to that natural release in which your head is moving, your body is widening and following your head? This frees up the vision."

A similar movement and awareness system, known formally as Functional Integration, was developed by the charismatic physicist, engineer, and bodyworker Moshe Feldenkrais (1904-1984). Feldenkrais work is a combination of body therapy, exercise, and movement instruction that seeks to reprogram the brain itself. As do Rolfers and Alexander teachers, Feldenkrais practitioners always look at the whole person and his or her patterns of action and movement.

According to veteran Feldenkrais practitioner Elizabeth Beringer, "It's relatively common that people experience vision improvement when doing Feldenkrais exercises, even if that wasn't their goal. But we would never look at someone's eyes separately from the rest of their body." Feldenkrais taught that the eyes are anchored within the whole body musculature, as well as within the life context of the individual—personal history, accidents, athletic activities, profession, and recreations.

"You cannot separate how somebody uses her neck and how much tension and tightness there is in the neck, with how she uses her eyes. If you simply put your palm on the back of your neck, then turn your eyes left then right, you can feel the neck muscles contracting," Beringer says.

Feldenkrais demonstrated that when a person learns to move skillfully, it has an impact on every aspect of self-image and motor behavior, including the eyes. One of Feldenkrais's most celebrated cases was a woman who had lost her vision from a cerebral hemorrhage. Feldenkrais was able to guide this patient out of "the jungle of the brain" brought on by the stroke, allowing her to walk and see again. As Karl Pribram, M.D., the renowned Stanford University neurosurgeon once said, "Feldenkrais is not just pushing muscles around, but changing things in the brain itself."

In the Feldenkrais model, lasting change takes place through the central nervous system. In this view, an emphasis on relaxing the eye muscles to improve vision, for instance, is only a start. It's difficult to reduce the normal state of continuous slight tension in muscle tissue and stress in one area of the body system, explains Beringer, "unless you reduce it throughout the system." You can't make a fist without contracting your arms and shoulders, argues Beringer. In the same way, if you think you can relax only the eye muscles but keep your neck, back, and breathing tight, you'll find it doesn't work.

Thus, an individual may consult Beringer for a back problem and be surprised to find in the course of work that his vision improves. Most people come in with a host of conditions related to vision, Beringer notes. "Moreover, working with the eyes is a particularly powerful way to affect all aspects of a person's functioning."

Unlike the Alexander Technique, the 800 U.S. practitioners of the Feldenkrais Method don't insist on a set number of sessions. Instruction is available on an individually tailored basis, in group classes, and privately at home through the use of practice tapes.

In his book of 12 core lessons, *Awareness Through Movement*, Feldenkrais included a series of exercises that illustrate how eye movements coordinate body movements and how they are linked to the movement of the neck muscles as well. He said, "Note the important role the eyes play in coordinating the musculature of the body; it is even greater than that of the neck muscles. Similarly, the muscles of the eyes and neck have a decisive influence on the manner in which the neck muscles contract."

Relaxing for Better Vision

The ancient Indian practice of hatha yoga is another discipline that embodies a number of the underlying principles of holistic bodywork. According to yoga teacher Richard Miller, "Generally, we look to see if body or neck muscles are tight and stressed. If they are, the eyes suffer. We look at the different energetic systems—kidneys, liver, gall bladder, pancreas, stomach—because these all have an impact on the eyes. Different poses work for these systems energetically and reduce systemic stress. If tension is the problem behind your reduced eyesight, you'll see results after a week of practicing these poses. If it's more than simple ocular muscle tension, if you practice the poses and breathwork, you should get changes within two months."

Miller makes his predictions from personal experience. He was once farsighted and required reading glasses. After a period of practicing a regime of specific poses, he no longer needed them. The best combination for a person starting a vision recovery program, says Miller, is to first get an energetic diagnosis from a whole systems discipline such as Chinese medicine. If the vision problem seems to be primarily from muscular tension, exercises including yoga and Bates may reverse the vision problem. If the problem is more systemic, then he recommends a combination of yoga, herbal remedies, and energetics, such as acupuncture.

Do the following exercises without correctional lenses.

EYE PURIFICATION. Traditionally, this a cleansing exercise whereby you gaze with eyes closed at the tip of your nose. It's an approach with many variations. For instance, in a semi-dark room gaze without blinking at an object such as a candle until the eyes begin to produce tears. Here the staring is therapeutically useful but only for the duration of the exercise. Afterwards, return to frequent blinking and non-staring. As a variation, hold a pencil with words inscribed on its shank as close to your eyes as possible while still legible. Focus, then bring it in a couple of inches closer. Focus again and continue bringing it closer to your eyes in small increments.

ARM-RAISE. Stand with your feet parallel and slightly spread apart and your knees gently flexed. Allow your arms to hang loosely at your sides and close your eyes and mouth. As you slowly, evenly inhale through the nose, gradually raise your arms to a position straight up over your head, as if you're pointing to the sky. Don't lift your head but keep it facing straight ahead. As you slowly exhale through the nose, lower your arms to their original position at your side. Practice this exercise six times.

THE BRIDGE. Lie comfortably flat on the floor on a yoga mat or thick blanket, with your legs about six inches apart and your arms extended palms down parallel with your torso. On the inhale lift the hips and back off the floor while keeping the arms flat against the floor. On the exhale, gently lower your body. Repeat this twice. For a variation, assume the original position but raise and bend your knees and put your feet flat on the floor close to your buttocks. On the inhale, raise both arms above your head (along the floor) as if pointing. While doing this, lift your buttocks and lower back off the floor. Hold for a few seconds, then gently lower on the exhale.

FLOOR-TOUCH. While standing with your legs six inches apart, inhale as you raise both arms above your head. On the exhale bend your torso forward, bending the knees slightly, so that your forehead approaches your kneecaps and the fingers approach the floor. Hold a few seconds. On the exhale, return to the original standing position. Relax and then repeat six times. After the sixth repetition, lower your arms to your sides as you exhale.

HALF SHOULDER STAND. Lie on the floor on your back with your knees raised and your feet close to your buttocks. Position your arms parallel to your torso, palms down. On the exhale, press your palms against the floor while lifting the legs back over your head until they're at a 45 degree angle to the floor. Prop your buttocks and lower back with your palms, but keep your elbows on the floor. Your weight in this pose is carried mainly by the arms and upper back. Remain in this pose for a minute, if that's comfortable without straining, and breathe calmly. Then, slowly and gently lower your legs by rolling your spinal column out on the floor. When your buttocks are on the ground again, bring the legs forward and down in smooth increments until they rest on the floor. This exercise is intensely invigorating.

FULL SHOULDER STAND. This one is even more beneficial to the eyes, brain, and neck in terms of increased blood circulation, though it shouldn't be practiced if you have any neck problems or chronic neck tension. It may help to perform this pose with the assistance of a partner. Position yourself as for the half shoulder stand, then slowly raise both legs to a vertical position so that the feet point towards the ceiling. Hold for 5-10 seconds, then gradually lower your back and legs as in the half shoulder stand.

The headstand is somewhat more difficult than the full shoulder stand and can be especially beneficial for vision problems. Mastery of the head stand is worth the effort, advises Miller, because it bathes the brain in increased blood and nerve flow for the following 24 hours. Like the full shoulder stand, it's not recommended for anyone with neck problems or chronic neck tension, and is best taught by an experienced yoga instructor.

SLANT BOARD. This is not a classical yoga posture, but rather a clever improvisation on the relaxing "corpse pose." Take a broad, thick plank and set one end atop an 18-inch brick or stack of books. Lie down on the plank with your head at the lower end, your arms at your sides. While breathing with attention, practice the eye stretches described in Step One.

KNEELING IMMERSION. This pose comes highly recommended by vision author Christopher Markert for increasing blood circulation around the eyes. Assume a kneeling position on the floor. Slowly lower your torso from the waist up until your forehead touches the floor in front of your knees. Extend your arms straight out behind you, approaching your feet. Hold for several inhale-exhale cycles as you notice the increased blood supply to your brain and eyes, then resume your original kneeling position. Next, fill a large shallow bowl, about 18 inches wide and 6 inches deep, with cool, clean water. Repeat the steps just described, but this time lower your head into the bowl of water, submerging your forehead and open eyes. Roll your open eyes circularly and blink frequently for a minute or so.

General aerobic exercises are often overlooked in the context of a vision recovery program. Consider the benefits of jogging, bicycling, swimming, skipping rope, calisthenics, tennis, and regular brisk walking. "The physical conditioning most relevant to visual training involves aerobic exercises to strengthen the cardiovascular system, and balancing exercises to improve body awareness, coordination, and timing," comment Ann and Townsend Hoopes, who followed their own good advice when they undertook to improve their vision.

The Hoopeses' highest recommendation, and one I personally concur with, is brisk walking. "Whatever their differences on physical conditioning, however, all visual-training optometrists appear to agree wholeheartedly that walking is the ideal exercise for improving vision and balancing the body/mind system," they note. While walking briskly without corrective lenses, you perceptually consume large volumes of space. You also benefit in terms of balance, coordination, use, and peripheral awareness.

Step Six: The Food and Light Nutrients

Feed your body and your eyes a diet—of foods, supplements, and light—for optimum visual health.

The process of vision is nutritionally expensive. The visual system and brain combined, while representing only 2 percent of body weight, require 25 percent of your food energy intake. Obviously, it's crucial to support vision improvement gains with nutritional and dietary practices. What do your eyes like to eat? In particular, vitamins A, B complex, C, D, and E, and the minerals calcium, zinc, and chromium. The visual system also feeds on light, an important nutrient for not only seeing well but staying healthy in other ways. And according to a controversial vision therapy, your eyes also feed on color.

As we consider nutrients, whether in the form of food or electromagnetic energy, remember that people have unique requirements. Foods, supplements, and exposure to sunlight should be adjusted to your biochemical condition and state of health. In addition, nutrients that help to improve vision also affect overall health and should be considered in relation to other bodily needs.

The Vision Vitamins and Minerals

To determine a safe and effective level of supplementation for the vitamins and minerals to follow, it's helpful to look at the levels supplied by a variety of "insurance formula" supplements. These are the supplements, usually taken as a pill or capsule up to six times a day, that are formulated to provide greater protection against marginal deficiencies than even the Recommended Dietary Allowances (RDAs) established by the federal National Research Council. Rainbow Light's Complete Nutritional System, Schiff's Single Day, New Chapter's Every Man, and Trigo's Natural

Timed Energy are some of the many insurance formulas available in natural foods stores. Most such formulas cover all eleven vitamins, four minerals, and three trace elements for which the government has determined there are RDAs. The supplements provide nutrient levels that range from the exact amount of the RDA to many times the RDA. Almost all nutritionists consider such insurance formulas safe for daily consumption by anyone.

VITAMIN A. Folk wisdom has long linked vitamin A with good vision, particularly the ability to see well at night, but it wasn't until the late 1950s that scientists began to understand that the chemistry of vision actually hinges on vitamin A. You may recall from the discussion of the eye's anatomy that vitamin A is a prime component of rhodopsin, the active pigment of the retina's photoreceptor rods. Vitamin A from the foods we eat migrates to the rods within the retina. It then binds with a colorless protein molecule called opsin, and in the form of rhodopsin permeates the light-sensitive tip of each cell within the rod. When a photon of light strikes the rhodopsin molecule, vitamin A breaks loose from its chemical bond with opsin and creates an electrical disruption that leads to perception. This single photochemical transformation—the release of vitamin A from its opsin molecular bond—is the core event in seeing.

Thus, not surprisingly, a vitamin A deficiency typically produces vision or eye problems such as poor rapid dark adaptation, pink or inflamed eyelids, and dryness of the cornea. Nutritionists estimate that as many as one in five Americans exhibit the visual indicators of a chronic vitamin A deficiency.

Among the richest dietary sources of vitamin A are fish-liver oil and animal products such as calf's liver. Vitamin A is also available in supplement form. Such concentrated sources should be approached with care, however, because vitamin A (along with D, E, and K) is a fat-soluble vitamin. More easily than the water-soluble vitamins, fat-soluble vitamins can build up to toxic levels in the body. Optimal requirements for vitamin A vary widely, and what is beneficial for one person may be harmful to another. Signs of vitamin A toxicity include blurred vision, persistent headaches, nausea, hair loss, and skin lesions. Fortunately, a safer form of vitamin A exists.

There are a number of natural pigments called carotenoids in some plants and animals that, when consumed, are processed by the liver into vitamin A. The most effective such vitamin A "precursor" is beta carotene, which does not have a tendency to accumulate in the body nor cause toxic reactions. Carrots are a well-known source of beta carotene, but it's found in even richer amounts in most green leafy vegetables, such as kale, spinach, collards, and mustard greens. The darker and more intense the green, the greater the concentration of beta carotene. In addition to carrots, other orange-colored vegetables and fruits, including apricots, nectarines, pumpkins, cantaloupes, yams, and squash are also high in beta carotene. Edible sea vegetables such as nori are also good sources.

The RDAs for vitamin A are now calculated using units of "retinol equivalents." As with most RDAs, a range of values is provided: 375 RE for infants, 800-1,000 RE for adult men and women, and 1,300 RE for lactating women. The formula for translating RE to International Units (IU), the value still used by most food and vitamin manufacturers, is complex but suffice it to say that the RDA for adults is in the range of 4,000-5,000 IU, while the insurance formulas typically provide 10,000 IU.

VITAMIN B COMPLEX. Within the 15-member vitamin B complex, thiamine (B_1), riboflavin (B_2), B_6, and B_{12} are potentially important to vision.

Too little thiamine in the diet results in burning or dry eyes, unclear or double vision, pain behind the eyeball, and involuntary eye movements. Prominent dietary sources of thiamine include whole grains, beans, some seeds and nuts, and seafood.

The thiamine RDAs for adults range from 1.0-1.5 mg, with higher amounts recommended for those who consume excessive amounts of coffee, tea, or alcohol. Levels in insurance formulas range from 45-75 mg.

Symptoms of a riboflavin deficiency include burning or bloodshot eyes, conjunctivitis, eye fatigue, sensitivity to light, pupil dilation, twilight blindness, and dark spots in the field of vision. Undernourished pregnant women, for example, during the final months of term, often experience burning sensations in the eyes, excess watering, and failing vision, all of which are helped by large doses of riboflavin. In some instances as little as 5 mg of riboflavin have alleviated symptoms. In one study of 47 patients with visual problems, several patients reported relief of symptoms after only one day of taking 15 mg of riboflavin. After nine months, six patients who had begun the program with cataracts had "reabsorbed" them and enjoyed normal lens function.

The richest dietary sources of riboflavin include brewers yeast and organ meats, though it is also well represented in dairy products, fish, whole grains, dried beans and peas, sunflower seeds, and leafy green vegetables. The riboflavin RDA is 1.2-1.7 mg, while insurance supplements range from about 50-75 mg.

Nutritionists have yet to come to a definitive view on the role of vitamin B_6 and vision, but they suspect the vitamin may regulate eye pressure (and thus help prevent glaucoma) and inhibit cataracts. The RDA is 1.6-2.0 mg and insurance formulas offer supplementation in the range of 50-75 mg.

A deficiency of vitamin B_{12} may lead to such neurologic problems as memory loss, disorientation, fatigue, and disruptions of gait and walking. These conditions can in turn impair the visual process, causing difficulty in focusing, a loss of central vision, and a general dimming of vision. Excessive cigarette smoking destroys B_{12}, so if you smoke and wear glasses, you probably need more B_{12}.

Most nutritionists agree that B_{12} is not synthesized by humans, though other animals do have microorganisms in their intestines that synthesize B_{12}. These bacteria (and some fungi) are the ultimate source of most B_{12} for humans. Whether there are reliable plant sources of this vitamin is a controversial topic. Some studies do indicate that the vitamin has been found in measurable amounts on fermented soybean products such as tempeh, single-cell proteins such as yeasts and the algae product spirulina, and certain sea vegetables. Though the reliability of such vegetarian sources is suspect, the human body needs only minute levels of B_{12} and also apparently does a good job of storing the vitamin. Most nutritionists agree that deficiencies are rare, though one population that should be especially aware of the vitamin is long-term vegans (those who eat absolutely no meat, fish, eggs, or dairy products).

The B_{12} RDA for adults is 2 mcg, and insurance formulas offer 30-180 mcg.

Choline, which some nutritionists consider a B vitamin and others a lipid, is, with inositol, the prime constituent of lecithin. Lecithin is essential for the health of the myelin sheaths that comprise all nerve fibers, including the optic fibers of the eyes. Choline facilitates the transmission of nerve impulses and helps regulate liver and kidney function. Reliable sources include egg yolks, soybeans, cauliflower, and cabbage. The federal government has established no RDA for choline.

VITAMIN C. As nutritionists continue to plumb the versatility of vitamin C or ascorbic acid, it appears this nutrient is beneficial for a variety of conditions, including vision problems. The eye's sclera depends on vitamin C to maintain its normal structure through building collagen, a primary component of connective tissue. The eyes' vitamin C levels exceed that of any other bodily organ, and the vitamin C composition of the aqueous humor is 20 times higher than that of any other bodily fluid.

Cataract formation may begin when vitamin C levels in the lens become deficient. A prominent nutritional study done in the 1980s at Tufts University indicated that the lenses of patients with high levels of vitamin C were less likely to produce cataracts.

Studies suggest vitamin C may be useful not only to prevent glaucoma but to treat it. Considerable research demonstrates a direct link between low vitamin C intake and increased intraocular pressure, the precondition of glaucoma. In addition, vitamin C supplementation has proven beneficial in reducing dangerous levels of eye pressure as quickly as in six days with 2 grams daily intake. In another study, intraocular pressure was significantly lowered after a week's intake of 500 mg of ascorbic acid twice daily.

The RDA for vitamin C is 60 mg per day, although insurance supplements range from 150 to 1,000 mg. The staunchest advocates of vitamin C such as Linus Pauling take thousands of mg per day. Vitamin C is easily leached out of the body and toxicity levels have not yet been proven.

VITAMIN D AND CALCIUM. This vitamin/mineral combination may play an important role in vision improvement. A number of nutritional studies have linked childhood myopia with calcium deficiency. Also, in a study at Columbia University's College of Physicians and Surgeons, animals fed diets deficient in vitamin D and calcium developed reduced arterial circulation and numerous eye problems.

Ophthalmologist Arthur Knapp, M.D., of New York City, has successfully treated numerous cases of rapidly increasing myopia with vitamin D and calcium supplementation. In some cases acuity improved from 20/400 to 20/200. Knapp has also administered high doses of the vitamin D and calcium combination to patients suffering from various eye ailments, including corneal protrusion, detached retina, and glaucoma, and noted a significant improvement in many cases.

These nutrients are administered together because vitamin D is necessary for the assimilation of calcium, which is a prime ingredient in bones, teeth, and all collagen-bearing connective tissues and muscles, including the sclera of the eyes. The link between vitamin D, calcium, and nearsightedness appears to be a waterlogged sclera. If the fibrous tunic around the eye contains too much water, it's susceptible to intraocular pressure and elongation, the anatomical signature of myopia. The vitamin D and calcium combination helps to dehydrate the waterlogged sclera, allowing the tunic to resume its normal shape and reducing the myopia as well.

In the early 1980s optometrist Ben Lane of Lake Hiawatha, N.J., identified another crucial dietary link with nearsightedness. He started with the clinical observation that myopic children tend to be significantly deficient in dietary calcium. He found that compared to children with normal acuity, the diet of nearsighted children contains higher levels of refined, simple carbohydrates. Lane noted that these same children also consume three times more animal protein than the clear-seeing children.

A common consequence of such a diet is a deficiency of vitamins and minerals, including calcium and chromium, and an overabundance of the mineral phosphorous. High phosphorous levels have an adverse effect on calcium in the blood, resulting in a withdrawal of calcium from the scleral tissue and bones of the eyes, a weakening of scleral structure, and increased excitability of the ciliary muscles. The result is a distention and contraction of the sclera—and highly compromised acuity. Lane concluded that preventing nearsightedness in children and adolescents calls for adequate intake and absorption of the nutrients responsible for maintaining normal eyeball pressure and enhancing the strength of scleral collagen.

Most vitamin D is manufactured by the body as the result of a process that begins with the sun's rays striking the skin. The vitamin is also available through such foods as egg yolks, fatty fish, and milk. The RDA is the equivalent of 200-400 IU and the insurance formulas typically provide 100-400 IU. Individual requirements vary and this is one of the easier vitamins to overdose on, either by consuming too much of the vitamin or exposing the body to too much sun. Over time this can lead to the toxic condition hypercalcemia, characterized by elevated blood levels of calcium. The body responds to this condition by depositing calcium in blood vessels, heart, lungs, and internal organs, where it basically makes a nuisance of itself and gums up the works.

Dietary sources of calcium include dairy products, tofu, and some leafy green vegetables such as broccoli, collards, spinach, and turnip and mustard greens. The RDA for calcium is 800-1,200 mg, and the insurance formulas range all the way from 10 mg to 1,000 mg.

VITAMIN E. Vitamin E helps prevent aging by acting as an antioxidant. That is, it helps prevent important components of living tissue from being "burned up" by oxygen. Along with the trace mineral zinc, vitamin E can also affect how the body uses vitamin A. For instance, more than 600 IU of E daily can interfere with beta carotene absorption. On the other hand, nutritionists have established that vitamin E has positive effects on vision. It can help improve acuity, arrest macular degeneration, reverse presbyopia, and, in some instances, keep childhood myopia from getting any worse.

Vitamin E nourishes the connective tissues of the eyes, making them stronger and more resilient. This allows the eyes to better resist the effects of near-point work that threaten to elongate the eyeball and produce myopia. Vitamin E may also have a beneficial effect on amblyopia, cataracts, and eyestrain, as well as liver and kidney function.

Reliable dietary sources of vitamin E include whole grain cereals, eggs, raw wheat germ, vegetable oils (especially wheat germ, corn, cottonseed, and safflower), raw almonds, hazelnuts, roasted peanuts, Brazil nuts, lettuce, spinach, watercress, turnip greens, kale, peas, cucumber, and asparagus. The vitamin E RDA is now calculated as "tocopherol equivalents," but in terms of IU the range is approximately 8-10. Insurance formulas offer 75-410 IU.

ZINC. Vitamin A metabolism and absorption and thus the rapid dark adaptation required for night vision may be impaired by a deficiency in zinc. Insufficient levels of zinc have also been implicated in macular degeneration. In one study of 150 elderly patients, zinc supplementation of 100 mg twice daily with meals produced significantly less visual loss and no side effects. Another study revealed that people with poor night vision taking vitamin A supplements showed no improvement until 90 mg per day of zinc were added to their nutritional program.

Many animal and fish products are high in zinc. As with vitamin A adequate amounts of zinc can be derived from plants, though levels vary widely depending upon the soil in which the plants are grown. Some of the better vegetarian sources are usually wheat germ or bran, brown rice, almonds, walnuts, and nectarines.

RDAs for zinc range from 12-15 mg while insurance supplement formulas run 15-50 mg. When taken as a separate supplement, it's best that zinc be mixed with copper and selenium, since excess zinc may upset its balance with these other minerals.

CHROMIUM. This trace mineral is vital to how the body regulates its energy supplies. Since the eyes are a major consumer of body energy, a chromium deficiency that encourages a condition of low blood sugar may contribute directly to poor vision. Marginal chromium deficiencies may in fact be common among contemporary Americans, especially among those consuming a diet high in refined, processed foods. Also, chromium levels in the body are depleted by strenuous exercise, and they dramatically decline with age. One nutritional study revealed that nearsighted children had 66 percent less chromium than children with no vision problems.

Deficiencies in both chromium and calcium may be produced by excessive consumption of refined carbohydrates and simple sugars. That's because chromium is required for the conversion of foods into muscle energy. In the eye, chromium is needed to enable the ciliary muscles to absorb glucose, the fuel necessary for their focusing action. When chromium supplies are low, focusing requires more effort and may be compromised. This produces more intraocular pressure which can eventually produce the elongation of the eyeball associated with myopia.

Whole grain cereals, brewers yeast, and some herbs and spices (particularly black pepper and thyme) are among the best dietary sources of chromium. Refined white sugar and white flour products not only have extremely low levels but they tend to deplete body chromium. There is no RDA for chromium.

Eating and Your Eyes

In addition to being affected by levels of specific vitamins and minerals, eye health and visual performance can deteriorate or improve depending on the overall quality of the diet. For instance, though scientific studies are lacking on the role of highly refined diets and blood sugar levels in affecting vision, a link has been noticed by a number of vision therapists, including Robert-Michael Kaplan. His experience with students has led him to conclude that the eye muscle responsible for accommodative focusing is sensitive to fluctuations in blood sugar levels. He says that he's observed this directly in several visually distressed students, such as a man who hadn't worn his strong glasses for eight days and had witnessed a 30 percent leap in his vision fitness, until he overindulged in rich food at a restaurant one night during the program. "Within 30 minutes his vision fitness had dropped so much that his wife had to lead him by the arm from the restaurant," comments Kaplan. "The intake of certain foods by sensitive individuals seems to trigger a chemical change that is recorded by the eyes," he adds.

In this sense the eyes are a kind of dumping ground for all the mistakes of your diet, says Kaplan. The conduit is the blood, and the vitality of your blood is only as good as the ability of your kidneys and liver to protect you from ill-considered dietary choices. To keep the eyes energized with nutrient-rich blood, it's important not to overload your system with a steady diet of fatty and sugary foods, stimulants, and antibiotics.

Among the foods that promote the maximum performance of organs such as the liver and kidney are leafy green vegetables. Traditional Chinese healers, who use foods and herbs to manipulate certain "qualities" such as "heatness" and "dampness" associated with distressed organs, affirm the healing effects of chlorophyll. "The liver has a tendency to get overheated from too many chemical toxins, so it likes fresh green vegetables because the chlorophyll helps detoxify and cool the organ," explains Raymond Himmel. "I always recommend lots of green foods, such as spirulina or blue-green algae, and lots of cooked green vegetables, such as chard, kale, bok choy, and alfalfa sprouts," he says. "It's equally important to not overeat foods that aggravate the liver, such as chocolate, nut butters, alcohol, and rich butter and cheese sauces."

In conclusion, keep in mind that a wholesome diet promotes the optimum health of all bodily systems, not only the eyes. Also, if you've any doubt about your nutritional condition and what amounts of the vision-related nutrients you should take in the context of a comprehensive dietary plan, consult a qualified nutritionist for advice.

The Full-Spectrum Diet

The eyes receive light not only for vision but as an essential source of nutrition. Light provides both the information we "read" through our eyes as well as the eyes' "food." This means it's essential to understand what proper "light" nutrition for the eyes involves.

Light entering through the eyes is a vital nutrient specifically for the hypothalamus, pineal, and pituitary glands, which are specialized hormone control centers located in the brain. These glands affect the body's biological rhythms, metabolic and respiration rates, blood pressure, liver, kidney, and pancreas functions, immune response, and even emotional states. The hypothalamus "may be the single most important unit of the brain, standing as high command in maintaining harmony within the body," comments Liberman, author of the book *Light: Medicine of the Future*.

The pineal is the body's light meter, responsible for the circadian release of melatonin, a master hormone of vast importance. A deficiency of melatonin is directly implicated in Seasonal Affective Disorder or SAD, the "winter blues" common in northern climates. The pineal's effects on the rest of the body are so wide-ranging that, according to Liberman, "Not a single cell in the body can escape the influence of light striking the eyes. We truly are light bodies."

It's easy to take light for granted, but not all light is equally beneficial to our health. The source of the light can have a major impact on how it affects the body. Over eons humanity has adapted to natural light from the sun that is characterized by a certain spectral energy pattern. A profile of the color characteristics of natural sunlight, for instance, will show the relative energy levels of ultraviolet and the colors violet, blue, green, yellow, orange, and red. These energy bands will differ for light from artificial sources, such as incandescent or fluorescent bulbs. The latter, for instance, typically have much higher levels of energy in the yellow band of the light spectrum.

Light with "spikes" in certain energy bands not only affects how illuminated objects appear to us, but long-term exposure to it can lead to "spectrum deficiency" and "malillumination" health problems, according to light researcher Dr. John Ott, formerly director of the Environmental Health and Light Research Institute in Sarasota, Fla. Ott notes, for example, that a 1980 study found that prolonged exposure to strong, artificial cool-white illumination, such as from most fluorescent lights, resulted in high levels in the body of certain metabolic hormones related to stress as well as behavioral problems, physical and mental fatigue, and learning impairment.

Another concern is the level of ultraviolet radiation (UVR) in light. Since at least the 1920s medical researchers have been contending that, like the skin, the eyes need protection from exposure to excessive amounts of UVR. Ultraviolet radiation is normally absorbed by atmospheric ozone, but the ozone layer has been seriously depleted in recent decades. Thus, many doctors now say that overexposure to ultraviolet radiation is a major health concern of the 1990s.

It's also a widely held belief among most ophthalmologists, sunglass manufacturers, and health authorities today that UVR is capable of producing, even in ordinary dosages, cataracts, lens yellowing, irritation, and scleral and corneal inflammation. This contention, states Gerald Fishman, M.D., professor of ophthalmology at the University of Illinois College of Medicine in Chicago, is based on 20 years of "investigative data and critical observation and epidemiologic evidence. There's a lot of circumstantial evidence that chronic exposure to light, particularly to blue and ultraviolet light, can contribute to the development of cataracts and may be harmful to the retina." Certain bandwidths within the UVR family, says Fishman, seem implicated. Given this data, conclude Fishman and other ophthalmologists, the eyes should be shielded from UVR with sunglasses during most outdoor activities.

Not all researchers, however, are in agreement about the presumed ocular perils of UVR, nor are they in consensus about the unqualified advantages of routinely donning sunglasses for all outdoor activities. One such dissenting scientist is Ott, whose investigations have revealed intriguing links between full-spectrum lighting (either indoors from specially designed lights, or outdoors from unfiltered natural sunlight) and the recovery from various illnesses. Ott's work has also suggested tangible negative health factors from habitual wearing of sunglasses and from being exposed continually to limited-spectrum indoor lighting.

Ott likens sunlight to a food, noting that the greatest benefit usually comes from consuming the whole, integral product. Natural, full-spectrum sunlight is vital for the smooth functioning of key bodily functions, explains Ott. These include calcium absorption, hormonal secretion, emotional stability, dental health, and the preservation of biological circadian rhythms. UVR catalyzes the synthesis of vitamin D in the body and thus is essential for the formation of normal bones and teeth. It's not surprising, then, that Ott regards the current sunglass craze with medical misgivings. With some exceptions, Ott's program of light therapy calls for the removal from the face of all forms of glasses, clear and tinted, and any other impediments to the eyes' reception of the complete band of visible and UVR light. All UVR is not inimical to the human eye, concludes Ott.

Color as a Light Nutrient

The implication is that natural sunlight is a necessary nutrient for optimum health. More speculative is the possibility that specific colors, when beamed directly into the eyes, can reverse or cure certain diseases. This possibility was first explored in the 1930s by the American scientist Harry Riley Spitler, M.D. He demonstrated that pencil-thick beams of 31 variously colored lights projected directly onto the retina affected the nervous and endocrine systems and produced healthful outcomes, including improved vision. He termed this field of study syntonic optometry, from the psychological term for being in emotional equilibrium and responsive to the environment.

One of the leading spokespersons for syntonic optometry today is Liberman, who's president of the College of Syntonic Optometry in Aspen, Colorado. His experience with the field dates to 1974, when he was treating a seven-year-old girl whose vision was 20/200 in one eye and 20/20 in the other. "Using this approach I was able to improve the vision of the poorer eye to approximately 20/25 within 30 minutes," says Liberman, "and to 20/20 after five sessions." He has since successfully used syntonics to treat "an entire array" of vision problems, including nearsightedness, strabismus, and lazy-eye.

"It's like a cookbook approach that matches specific color frequencies with specific eye problems," says Liberman. "I've seen hundreds of patients become less nearsighted this way."

Recently Liberman has been looking into the possible effects of color on hyperactivity. Optometrists suspect that hyperactive children may have reduced peripheral vision, and that their incessant squirming and movement is an effort to see more of their world. Over a six-week period Liberman gave subjects light therapy four times a week in 20-minute sessions. The results were highly impressive. Average visual field increased by 300 percent, visual attention span was four times improved, visual memory seven times, and 75 percent of the children did better in schoolwork.

John Downing, O.D., founder of the Neurophotonic Institute in Mill Valley, California, has also found that colored light therapy can successfully treat learning disabilities, and adds that it is "highly effective" with hyperactivity, headaches, fatigue, and depression.

Improving Your Light Diet

Most Americans spend over 90 percent of their life indoors, a situation that puts them at risk for developing a "light deficiency." If you're one of these people, consider taking four practical steps to improve your light diet.

GET OUTDOORS FOR AT LEAST A SHORT PERIOD OF TIME EVERY DAY. A brisk walk, sans glasses or contacts, is a great invigorator for body and eyes. Try doing some of your usual indoor activities outdoors. Find a nice spot to read, meditate, or play a musical instrument. For those who have mostly forsaken the fine art of handwriting, modern technology has revived the writing-outdoors option with the proliferation of laptop computers. Even during the winter in northern climes, if you dress appropriately and find a sunny spot you can be comfortable long enough to give the eyes a nice natural light bath.

CURTAIL YOUR USE OF SUNGLASSES TO WHAT'S REALLY NECESSARY. Most of today's sunglasses not only reduce glare and brightness but filter out some portion of the UVR bandwidth. Overuse of sunglasses can make the eyes more light sensitive. And although the role of UVR in human health is complex and controversial, it's possible that at least some level of UVR may play a positive role in health.

That said, certainly sunglasses are sometimes necessary for health. A number of medical conditions call for sunglasses, and they are potentially important for the elderly, who are more susceptible to cataracts, those who have had cataract or other eye surgery, and people on medication such as oral contraceptives and acne medicines that increase one's sensitivity to light. People whose work or recreation exposes them to intense outdoor glare environments, whether it be from sailing, skiing, mountain climbing, or other conditions in which light transmittance is overwhelming, should also protect their eyes with sunglasses.

WHEN INDOORS, WORK OR PLAY NEXT TO A WINDOW OR UNDER A SKYLIGHT. In addition to being "full spectrum," natural light that streams indoors is often many times brighter than artificial light. Windows do block ultraviolet, but that's the one element of the natural light spectrum to which you don't want to be overexposed.

CONSIDER TAKING ADVANTAGE OF RECENT ADVANCES IN LIGHTING TECHNOLOGY. This is particularly important if you're still using conventional incandescent bulbs for your indoor light. There's an ongoing debate about the best form of artificial light, revolving mainly around such technical points as color temperature (whether a bulb provides a "warm" yellowish tone or a "cool" bluish tone typical of northern, mid-day sunlight), level of ultraviolet radiation, and color rendering index (how closely a light duplicates the visible spectrum of sunlight). After reviewing much of the data, I've determined that there are three progressively better options to conventional incandescents. Unfortunately, the choices are also progressively more expensive.

First, a color-corrected incandescent bulb (look for one that says it is made with neodymium or cobalt technology) is a slight improvement on a regular incandescent. A number of bulb manufacturers make such incandescents, sometimes calling them "full-spectrum" even though the bulbs' spectral curve is still somewhat distorted compared to that of natural light.

The second choice, a full-spectrum fluorescent lamp such as the Vita-Lite manufactured by the Duro-Test Corporation of North Bergen, N.J., has a high color rendering index and does have a spectral curve similar to that of sunlight. Such bulbs are considerable improvements on either conventional incandescents or fluorescents.

The third choice is one of the high-tech multi-bulb systems that has been developed for therapeutic use by sufferers of SAD. The size of a small suitcase and costing hundreds of dollars, these are powerful lights that, in addition to having favorable color and spectral attributes, also approach outdoor intensity levels. The Ott Light System, manufactured under license by the Lumax Corporation of Altoona, Penn., is an advanced model.

Step Seven: Establish Positive Visual Habits

Learn and adopt the positive lifestyle and work habits necessary for the long-term health of the visual system.

The steps we've recommended in this guide, from eye exercises to better nutrition, are suggestions for developing permanent, supportive habits to keep seeing naturally. As a final complement to these, you need to consider how lighting, posture, and the constant use of video display terminals, televisions, and other technologies affect your vision. This is especially crucial because so many Americans today do intensive near-point work that can wreak havoc on even the healthiest eyes.

Window-Gazing and Other Light Ideas

While natural light is unarguably the best, it's not always a practical option for many desk-bound professionals. For myself, I've set my computer next to a large window that looks out over a small lawn with woods beyond. Every few minutes I shift my gaze from my VDT screen to the outside world. I allow my eyes to shift or edge, and then relax a moment. Another large window to my left helps illuminate my office in daytime, while three lamps do the trick at night.

If you can't situate your computer or work area next to a window, you can imitate the therapeutic effects of window-gazing with a large wall picture of a natural scene. Find something large-featured, colorful, and tranquil, and allow your eyes to wander over it occasionally. Several broad-leaf plants close to your desk can also provide a surface area for edging and shifting. If even this is impossible, visualize a restful country scene. Also, take a few moments every hour to become aware of your peripheral visual space.

Above all, remember to blink a lot, breathe calmly and deeply, and pause every once in a while to palm your eyes. Habits to avoid are staring and holding the eyes rigidly fixed, and straining to see in visually difficult situations.

The previous chapter examined the quality of light coming from different bulbs. Equally important to visual health is the positioning and shading of the light source. One objective is to avoid glare, which causes you to have to struggle to read either the printed page or the VDT screen. You may want to experiment with different placements for computer, desk, or typewriter within the room to find the best spot to avoid reflected glare from windows, light fixtures, or bright walls. Also, you can put a glare screen or visor on the VDT. Ideally you want to cross-illuminate the work area, with the light sources about 3-4 feet from the printed material. I've found that adjustable-neck clamp-on lights positioned at each end of the desk work well at illuminating paper copy.

It's best to avoid great disparities between the relative levels of light at your VDT, for instance, and around your desk. The constant readjustments to changes in illumination or contrast tax the response of the retinas and can deplete vital stores of vitamin A. You may want to reduce the lighting in the immediate area around the VDT, or increase screen brightness.

Saving Back and Eyes with Better Posture

If you're a nine-year-old, maybe you can still get away with lying on your stomach in bed and reading by flashlight. Adults, on the other hand, often pay for even more mild forms of abuse (such as working hunched over a text lying flat on a desk) with backaches, neck problems, muscle strains, or worse. Vision professionals consistently advise that you read while sitting up, feet flat on the floor, in a relatively erect but muscularly unstressed position, preferably in a chair with firm back support. Edward G. Godnig, O.D., and John S. Hacunda, authors of *Computers and Visual Stress*, contend that it's best for the torso to incline about 20 degrees forward from the hips. The reading material should be held perpendicularly to the line of sight.

Vision expert Darrell Boyd Harmon of the University of Minnesota in Minneapolis studied the classroom conditions of thousands of schoolchildren who had developed visual difficulties and discovered that many of them suffered "postural deviations" far beyond what was normally tolerable. Contributing factors included window glare, flat-top desks that were set too low, and unreadable areas of the chalkboard. The result was that as children struggled to compensate for these poorly designed study conditions, they tilted their heads, thrust forward their chins, leaned to one side, or hunched over—all of which began to deteriorate their posture and vision. Harmon's work clearly demonstrated the direct feedback link between postural distortions and visual defects.

Whether reading or watching television in a chair, or working at a desk, it's best to avoid long periods of unchanged posture. Get up, stretch, and walk around at least briefly once an hour or so. For some people at work, this goes counter to an ethic that emphasizes optimal efficiency. (It may also go counter to a watchful supervisor's rules.) Recent work performance studies, however, support the view that frequent breaks and work intermissions not only greatly reduce eyestrain and visual fatigue, but improve overall performance, enhance concentration, and replenish physical and mental energy.

When you do get caught up in your work to such an extent that your eyes begin to blur and lose focus, try this remedial step. Shift your focus back and forth from a distant to near object, blink repeatedly, breathe with relaxation, and then palm for a few moments.

VDT: Vision Destroying Terminal?

VDT-based jobs are fast becoming commonplace for professions ranging from journalism to science to sales. And as any parent of a Nintendo-crazed adolescent can affirm, recreational use of computers and video games is rapidly accelerating. A conservative estimate is that over 40 million Americans use VDTs on a regular basis.

What these statistics do not tell us is how many of these millions develop visual stress symptoms directly related to their prolonged VDT work. Among the most common of these symptoms are eye focusing breakdown and eye coordination anomalies, according to Godnig and Hacunda. They contend that VDT eyestrain has become a "high tech health concern of our information society."

Eyestrain resulting from improper VDT use can take many and sometimes indirect forms. The more obvious, acute symptoms include eyestrain, blurred vision beyond close range, irritated or reddened eyes, headaches concurrent with VDT use, difficulties in shifting focus from screen to distant objects, double vision, alterations in color perception, reduced concentration, and discomfort with present eyeglass prescription. But among the more indirect VDT-stress symptoms noted by Godnig and Hacunda are otherwise unaccountable neck, shoulder, or back tension, stiffness, or pain; chronic fatigue, emotional irritability, or nervousness during VDT use; pain in the arms, wrists, or shoulders during use; and generally lowered visual efficiency and computing speed and accuracy. Any combination of these symptoms, if untreated and uncorrected, can only exacerbate an existing visual problem such as nearsightedness or farsightedness. Those with correctional lenses may find in a few months that they suddenly need stronger glasses. Those that don't wear glasses may find themselves suddenly needing them to do near-point work.

VDT-induced stress is a malady that affects more than a small group of full-time hackers and programmers, too. A 1985 study revealed that only 5-10 percent of American VDT users work under visually satisfactory workplace conditions. Another study undertaken in 1981 by the National Institute for Occupational Safety and Health reported that 84 percent of VDT users reported some level of general eyestrain, 67 percent reported a burning sensation in their eyes, and 40 percent complained of blurred vision.

Part of the remedy for VDT-induced visual stress is to redesign the work environment to minimize stress-producing conditions and to maximize the vision-enhancing conditions. One of the most important factors to consider is VDT viewing distance. Most people view their VDT screens from about 18-25 inches away. Vision experts differ in their recommendations, though they agree that 25 inches is too far. Harmon has worked out a precise calculation called "the Harmon distance" to determine how far to set a book or VDT screen during near-point work. He found that an ideal distance for near-point work is about the same distance as between the elbow and the middle knuckle of the middle finger. I'm 5'9" and for me, that's about 16 inches. The American Optometric Association recommends that the worker be 14-20 inches from the screen. Other experts say that the comfortable distance for reading is more like 12-16 inches, while Godnig and Hacunda put it at 20 inches. Work within this 12-20 inch range to see what feels best for you.

Another positive VDT habit is to keep screen and text about the same distance from the eyes and at about the same height and angle. The custom is to lay the book or document flat out on the desk under the screen or close to the body. This forces you to look down at the work and then up again to the screen, potentially stressing neck and eyes. Instead find a desk with a 20 degree incline or use an adjustable bookstand/manuscript holder positioned next to your VDT screen and raised to approximately the same height.

Some other recommendations for better vision habits while at the VDT include:

• Keep the line of sight from eyes to screen about 20 degrees below the horizontal.

• Match your paper and screen color, if possible, since frequent adjustment from dark screen to bright paper can cause eye strain.

• Maintain your VDT so that the screen is clean and the characters sharp. If possible adjust character size and focus for easiest viewing.

• Avoid using handwritten or hard-to-read source documents when working on a VDT.

• Keyboards should be detachable for optimum positioning, and light in color.

Better Vision Habits for Kids

A comprehensive vision undertaking for parents is to conserve the eyesight of their children. Parents in previous generations for the most part were unaware of steps for preserving visual health, and many of us regrettably experienced vision loss in childhood or adolescence as a result. The full range of recommendations and positive habits presented in this book can be offered in a better-vision program to children, whether from parents, schoolteachers, public health officials, nurses, or therapists.

Bates recommended the daily schoolroom use of simple test card or eye chart exercises to resolve childhood vision problems. People of all ages, he added, have "benefited by this treatment of errors of refraction by relaxation, but children usually, though not invariably, respond much more quickly than adults. If they are under twelve years of age, or even under sixteen, and have never worn glasses, the condition is usually eliminated in a few days, weeks, or months, and always within a year, simply by reading a test card every day."

According to Kavner, who's written a book on the topic called *Your Child's Vision*, the best service a parent can render his or her child's vision is early prevention of problems. This begins, ideally, during pregnancy. Unhealthful lifestyle choices during pregnancy, such as excessive alcohol or drug consumption, smoking, and unrelieved stress, can harm a child's vision before birth. Kavner also points to a number of key practices parents should keep in mind during the crucial early developmental years of a child.

LEARN HOW TO DIAGNOSE YOUR CHILD'S HEALTH AND DEVELOPMENT. Parents should pay attention to a child's motor skills, coordination and balance, speech, and depth perception, and learn how to compare these with standard developmental norms. Discrepancies or delays of more than 25 percent, says Kavner, may indicate budding visual and perceptual problems.

MAINTAIN THE BEST POSSIBLE HOME ENVIRONMENT FOR GROWTH. Kavner emphasizes the importance of offering love, providing sound nutrition, and controlling allergy-producing substances. For visual activities such as reading or watching television, parents should assure adequate glare-free lighting and encourage an erect, relaxed posture. He also suggests supervising regular "eye breaks" to have children do some of the simpler exercise and relaxation practices after every 20 minutes or so of reading or watching television.

WATCH YOUR CHILD CLOSELY RIGHT AFTER HE OR SHE EXPERI-

ENCES A TRAUMA OR CHILDHOOD DISEASE. "These periods of debilitation can interfere with completing critical phases of visual development," Kavner notes. For instance, strabismus can develop following a bout of measles and myopia following a prolonged fever or high-stress experience.

Part Three:
Take Charge of Your Vision

Your Personal Program for Seeing Better

As Bates pointed out, "Daily practice of the art of vision is necessary to prevent those visual lapses to which every eye is liable, no matter how good its sight may be ordinarily." This is the key to success in reclaiming your vision naturally. Over the past year, I've gained a far more comprehensive appreciation of the many components of the art of vision.

I've learned that the holistic, natural approach to vision improvement involves a great deal more than the occasional visit to an optometrist's office, even if it's to an innovative optometrist like Stern or Kaplan, or some other natural vision improvement teacher. I've come to understand how complex an aspect of my whole life and being is this question of good eyesight. This complexity starts with the eye, that marvellous instrument so precisely fine-tuned to nearly instantaneously receive, organize, and interpret millions of bits of light, but it hardly ends there.

To really understand vision, it's necessary to see it in context of not only the eyes, but the brain, the nervous system, hormonal functions, genetics, the liver, diet, behavior, work and play habits, psycho-emotional states, and more. The popular perception of vision as an isolated, detached function is inconsistent with the holistic approach to health and medicine in general. Natural healers of various backgrounds, whether acupuncturist or herbalist, would tend to agree that the quality and precision of your eyesight arises out of the constantly changing energetic status of your whole body/mind system.

Fortunately, the world of complementary, alternative, and natural holistic medicine has numerous self-care options, from acupressure massage and breathing exercises to herbs and postural analysis. For those who resolve to improve their vision, the tools of natural medicine present themselves as allies.

Every individual is biochemically unique. Thus, any recommendation for natural, holistic vision improvement can only be made conditionally. The advice needs to be judged by you, the reader, and put to use selectively, according to your need, condition, temperament, and general inclinations. For some this may mean eye exercises, diet, and yoga. For others, introspective work, special glasses, and herbs. There may be some readers of this book with the time and commitment to try almost all of the possible therapies. If you're not one of these people, don't feel discouraged. Do what you're comfortable with, approach it with an attitude of having fun, and give it your best shot.

I'm convinced that the decision to *want* to see better is the cornerstone of any vision improvement program. Then it's only a matter of identifying the physical and psycho-emotional obstacles that stand in the way of enhanced eyesight and calling on any of a host of effective, natural, selfcare options. How long it takes and how far you make it back to 20/20 is entirely variable. My own case of extreme nearsightedness has improved markedly since I began to explore vision improvement strategies, and it's continuing to improve. But I will not consider my work a failure, and my eyesight abominable, even if I can never correct it to 20/20. Sharp acuity is a worthwhile goal, but as we've seen vision is much more than that.

The 20/20 standard, in fact, may be a misleading and unnecessary goal. What is a goal worth striving for is better visual performance, visual skills encompassing all the aspects of healthy eyesight—peripheral awareness, accommodative flexibility, binocular convergence and teaming, depth perception, rapid dark adaptation, eye-hand coordination, visual reaction time, eye tracking, and more. Though my acuity is still less than it could be, I'm now noticeably more comfortable, relaxed, and open with my seeing. The quality of my seeing, the way I approach the act of seeing, and how I practice the art of vision—all of these have become far healthier and more positive than I had thought possible, certainly after 33 years of the unexamined habit of wearing glasses.

I'm reminded that the goal, according to John Selby, is not to further condition the eyes. It is to free them through coming to a better understanding of the "intimate interplay between your eyes and the rest of your being." At the heart of this growth, says Selby, is the fact that "your brain knows how healthy vision functions. You were born with the natural ability to see clearly." With practice, it is indeed possible to reclaim this natural ability.

Resources for Natural Vision Improvement

Organizations and Practitioners

American Chiropractic Association, 1701 Clarendon Blvd., Arlington, VA 22209; (703) 276-8800. Information and practitioner referrals.

American Optometric Association, Communications Center, 243 North Lindbergh Blvd., St. Louis, MO 63141; (314) 991-4100; fax (314) 991-4101. Conventional eye care and optometric information and statistics, educational materials, and practitioner referrals.

Bastyr College of Natural Health Sciences, 144 N.E. 54th, Seattle, WA 98105; (206) 523-9585. Naturopathic books, educational materials, and practitioner referrals.

Bob Corey and Associates, P.O. Box 73, Merrick, NY 11566; (516) 485-5544. Full-spectrum fluorescent Vita-Lites.

Cambridge Institute for Better Vision, Martin Sussman, Director, 65 Wenham Rd., Topsfield, MA 01983; (508) 887-3883. Self-help training program, tapes, consultations, seminars, and books.

Center for Self Healing, Meir Schneider, Director, 1718 Taraval St., San Francisco, CA 94116; (415) 665-9574. Books, seminars, audio and video tapes, private therapy, and training programs in natural vision improvement and self-healing.

College of Syntonic Optometry, Jacob Liberman, O.D., President, P.O. Box 4058, Aspen, CO 81612. Information and training on light, color, and health.

Feldenkrais Resource Catalog, P.O. Box 2067, Berkeley, CA 94702; (800) 765-1907. Products, tapes, books, and practitioner referrals.

Feldenkrais Guild, P.O. Box 489, Albany, OR 97321; (503) 926-0981. Practitioner referrals.

Flower Essence Society, P.O. Box 459, Nevada City, CA 95959; (916) 265-9163. Flower essences, educational materials, and practitioner referrals.

Janet Goodrich, Crystal Waters Permaculture Village, MS-16, Maleny, Queensland 4552, Australia; (74) 944657; fax (74) 944673. U.S. office: Natural Vision Improvement, 1032 Irving St., Suite 233, San Francisco,

CA 94122; (415) 386-1550. Books, tapes, seminars, and training in natural vision improvement.

International Institute for Bioenergetic Analysis, 144 East 36th St., New York, NY 10016; (212) 532-7742. Books by Alexander Lowen, training programs, and practitioner referrals.

Meridian Traditional Herbal Products, 44 Linden St., Brookline, MA 02146; (800) 356-6003. Traditional Chinese patent medicines.

Natural Vision International, Ltd., P.O. Box 157, Manitowoc, WI 54221; (800) 255-4715; fax (414) 793-2425. Pinhole glasses, books, and natural vision training programs.

North American Society of Teachers of the Alexander Technique, P.O. Box 3992, Champaign, IL 61826; (217) 359-3529. Practitioner referrals.

Optometric Extension Program Foundation and Vision Extension, Inc., 2912 South Daimler St., Suite 100, Santa Ana, CA 92705; (714) 250-0846. Journals, pamphlets, vision products, seminars, training, information on behavioral optometry, and practitioner referrals.

Rolf Institute of Structural Integration, P.O. Box 1686, Boulder, CO 80306; (303) 449-5903. Practitioner referrals.

Seeing Beyond 20/20, Robert-Michael Kaplan, O.D., M.Ed., 3236 West 7th Ave., Vancouver, B.C., Canada V6K 2A2; (604) 737-2043; fax (604) 737-6866. Vision improvement product catalog, phone consultations, certified teacher trainings, and books.

Cathy Stern, O.D., Brookline Vision Associates, 56 Harvard St., Brookline, MA 02146; (617) 277-7754. Behavioral optometry consultations and examinations.

Books

The Art of Seeing by Aldous Huxley, Creative Arts Book Company, 1982, 147 pages, paperback, $7.95.

The Bates Method for Better Eyesight Without Glasses by William H. Bates, M.D., Henry Holt & Co., 1981, 200 pages, paperback, $7.95.

Better Sight Without Glasses by Harry Benjamin, Thorsons/HarperCollins, 1984, 96 pages, paperback, $4.95.

Do You Really Need Glasses? by Dr. Marilyn B. Rosanes-Berrett,

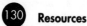

Pulse/Station Hill Press, 1990, 149 pages, paperback, $10.95.

Dr. Friedman's Vision Training Program by Edward Friedman, O.D., with Kalia Lilow, Bantam, 1983, 237 pages, paperback, $6.95.

Help Yourself to Better Sight by Margaret Darst Corbett, Wilshire Book Co., 1949, 217 pages, paperback, $7.00.

Natural Vision Improvement by Janet Goodrich, Ph.D., Celestial Arts, 1985, 218 pages, paperback, $14.95.

Seeing Beyond 20/20 by Robert-Michael Kaplan, O.D., Beyond Words Publishing, 1987, 218 pages, paperback, $12.95.

Seeing Well Again Without Your Glasses by Christopher Markert, C.W. Daniel Co., 1981, 123 pages, hardcover, $10.95.

Self-Healing: My Life and Vision by Meir Schneider, Arkana/Viking Penguin, 1987, 190 pages, paperback, $8.95.

Stress and Vision by Elliott B. Forrest, O.D., Optometric Extension Program Foundation, 1988, 318 pages, hardcover, $35.00.

Suddenly Successful: How Behavioral Optometry Helps You Overcome Learning, Health, and Behavior Problems by Hazel Richmond Dawkins, Dr. Ellis Edelman, and Dr. Constantine Forkiotis, Optometric Extension Program Foundation, 1991, 304 pages, hardcover, $22.95.

Total Vision by Richard S. Kavner, O.D., and Lorraine Dusky, Kavner Books, 1978, 264 pages, paperback, $9.95.

20/20 Is Not Enough by Dr. Arthur S. Seiderman and Dr. Steven E. Marcus, Alfred A. Knopf, 1989, 196 pages, hardcover, $18.95.

Vision: A Holistic Guide to Healing the Eyesight by Joanna Rotté, Ph.D., and Koji Yamamoto, Japan Publications, 1986, 152 pages, paperback, $14.95.

The Visual Handbook: The Complete Guide to Seeing More Clearly by John Selby, Element Books, 1987, 192 pages, paperback, $12.95.

Your Child's Vision: A Parent's Guide to Seeing, Growing, and Developing by Richard S. Kavner, O.D., Fireside/Simon & Schuster, 1985, 250 pages, paperback, $8.95.

About the Author

One of America's most prominent natural health journalists, Richard Leviton is the author of more than 75 feature articles for national publications in recent years. Currently a senior writer for *Yoga Journal* and a contributor to *East West/Natural Health*, he's been actively engaged both as businessman and journalist in the fields of natural foods and health since the mid-1970s. Formerly he was editor/publisher of *Soyfoods Magazine*, an international journal for commercial soyfoods entrepreneurs. His natural health articles have been widely reprinted in the U.S., Canada, Germany, Switzerland, Israel, and Australia. Leviton is also author of *The Imagination of Pentecost*, forthcoming in late 1992 from Anthroposophic Press.

Index

hand massage, 78-79
Refraction, 9
  illustration of, 14-15
  variability of, 21
Reich, Wilhelm, 62, 66, 68
Relaxation, 21
  exercises, 32-34
Retina, 6-9, 102
Retinal disease, 16
Rhodopsin, 8-9, 82, 102
Riboflavin, 103-104
Rocking the pelvis exercise, 63-64
Rods, 7-8, 82, 102
Rolf, Ida, 91
Rolfing, 91-93

Sclera, 5, 105, 106
Seasonal Affective Disorder (SAD),
  111, 116
Self assertion exercise, 72
Self hypnosis, 68-69
Seven Steps program, summary of,
  29-30
Shifting, 8, 13
  exercises, 36-38
Short swing exercise, 37-38
Shoulder and neck self massage, 77-
  78
Slant board exercise, 99
Snellen, Hermann, 11
  eye chart, 11-12, 24
  eye chart exercise, 36
Subluxation, 88-89
Sunglasses, 112-115
Sunlight, 111-113
Sunning, 33
Swinging ball exercise, 41

Taoist arch exercise, 64-65
Tear glands, 5
Therapeutic lenses, 45, 47-51
Thiamine, 103
Thumb fusion exercise, 40
Thumb zooming exercise, 35-36
Trampoline vision training, 57

Tromboning exercise, 35
Tunnel vision, 17

Ultraviolet radiation, 111-113, 115

Video display terminals, 117-121
Vision, functions of, 11-14
  common problems, 14-17
  structuralist vs. functional
    approach to, 28-29
  whole person approach to, 10,
    26, 46, 58
Visualization and imagination exer-
  cises, 41-43
Vitamin A, 8-9, 102-103, 118
Vitamin B complex, 103-105
Vitamin B6, 104
Vitamin B12, 104-105
Vitamin C, 105-106
Vitamin D, 106-107, 113
Vitamin E, 107-108
Vitreous humor, 6-7

Walking, 99-100
Watching the ball exercise, 34-35
Whipping exercise, 35

Yardstick fusion exercise, 40
Yawning exercise, 34
Yoga, 74, 79-81, 87, 91, 96-99

Zinc, 108

The Natural Health Bookshelf

Shop from home for the best guides to natural foods, holistic health, and whole foods cooking.

Order now toll-free: (800) 876-1001 Mon-Fri 9am-5pm EST. Visa and MasterCard accepted. Or order directly by mailing check or money order to Natural Health Books, P.O. Box 1200, 17 Station St., Brookline Village, MA 02147. Include $3.00 postage and handling for first book and $0.50 for each additional book.

Quick and Natural Rice Dishes: The 75 Most Popular Recipes from 20 Years of Natural Health Magazine from the Editors of Natural Health, 128 pages, paperback, $8.95

The Bread Book: A Natural, Whole-Grain Seed-to-Loaf Approach to Real Bread by Thom Leonard,110 pages, paperback, $8.95

Childbirth Wisdom: From the World's Oldest Societies by Judith Goldsmith, 291 pages, paperback, $10.95

Sweet & Natural Desserts: Wholesome, Sugar- and Dairy-Free Treats from the Editors of Natural Health, 120 pages, paperback, $8.95

Shopper's Guide to Natural Foods: A Consumer's Guide to Buying and Preparing Foods for Good Health from the Editors of Natural Health, 224 pages, paperback, $12.95

Meetings with Remarkable Men and Women from the Editors of Natural Health, 296 pages, paperback, $12.95

Fighting Radiation & Chemical Pollutants with Foods, Herbs, & Vitamins by Steven R. Schechter, N.D., 312 pages, paperback, $9.95

The Essential Movements of T'ai Chi by John Kostias, 169 pages, paperback, $11.95

Natural Childcare from the Editors of Natural Health, 216 pages, paperback, $10.95

Whole World Cookbook from the Editors of Natural Health, 140 pages, paperback, $6.95